Spanish for Veterinarians

A Practical Introduction

Second Edition

Spanish for Veterinarians

Veterinarians

A Practical Introduction

Second Edition

Bonnie Frederick
Juan Mosqueda

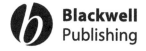

Blackwell
Publishing

Bonnie Frederick, PhD, is a professor of Spanish at Texas Christian University, Fort Worth, Texas. Her special area of research is women's culture and literature in Hispanic America.

Juan Mosqueda, MVZ, PhD, is a veterinarian working at the Centro Nacional de Investigacion Disciplinaria en Parasitología Veterinaria in Jiutepec, Morelos, Mexico. His special area of research is babesiosis.

Drs. Mosqueda and Frederick also wrote this book's companion volume, *Spanish for Animal Scientists and Food Animal Producers*, published by Blackwell.

Blackwell Publishing Professional
2121 State Avenue, Ames, Iowa 50014, USA

Orders: 1-800-862-6657
Office: 1-515-292-0140
Fax: 1-515-292-3348
Web site: www.blackwellprofessional.com

Blackwell Publishing Ltd
9600 Garsington Road, Oxford OX4 2DQ, UK
Tel.: +44 (0)1865 776868

Blackwell Publishing Asia
550 Swanston Street, Carlton, Victoria 3053, Australia
Tel.: +61 (0)3 8359 1011

Authorization to photocopy items for internal or personal use, or the internal or personal use of specific clients, is granted by Blackwell Publishing, provided that the base fee is paid directly to the Copyright Clearance Center, 222 Rosewood Drive, Danvers, MA 01923. For those organizations that have been granted a photocopy license by CCC, a separate system of payments has been arranged. The fee code for users of the Transactional Reporting Service is ISBN-13: 978-0-8138-0687-7/2008.

First edition, 2000
Second edition, 2008

Library of Congress Cataloging-in-Publication Data
Frederick, Bonnie.
  Spanish for veterinarians / Bonnie Frederick, Juan Mosqueda. – 2nd ed.
      p. cm.
  ISBN-13: 978-0-8138-0687-7 (alk. paper)
  ISBN-10: 0-8138-0687-9 (alk. paper)
1. Spanish language–Conversation and phrase books (for medical personnel)   I. Mosqueda, Juan.   II. Title.

  PC4120.M3F74 2008
  468.3′421024636–dc22

                                                                              2007049159

The last digit is the print number: 9 8 7 6 5 4 3 2 1

Contents

CHAPTER *5*

How Long Has the Cow Had a Fever?   33

CHAPTER *6*

The Past and Accidents   41

CHAPTER *7*

Telling People What to Do   49

CHAPTER *8*

Taking a Clinical History   57

CHAPTER *9*

The Diagnostic Exam   61

CHAPTER *10*

Cattle   67

CHAPTER *11*

Horses   75

CHAPTER *12*

Sheep and Goats 79

CHAPTER *13*

Swine 83

CHAPTER *14*

Dogs and Cats 87

CHAPTER *15*

Exotic Pets 93

APPENDIX

Registration Forms 99

Preface

This book is an introduction to the Spanish specific to veterinary medicine, and is not intended to make you a fluent Spanish speaker. Instead, it is designed to prepare you for the clinical conversations between a vet and a client. After studying these chapters, you will not be able to argue politics or discuss poetry. However, you will be able to ask what the animal's symptoms are and how long it has had the problem. Moreover, you'll be able to understand the gist of the client's answer. If you approach this study with that practical goal in mind, you should be able to learn a working Spanish fairly rapidly.

Because the aims of this book are so specific and practical, many elements of the Spanish language are not included. For example, you won't find the conditional verbs here. Even though they're lovely verbs, they aren't essential to the vet–client interaction, which depends mainly on present-tense and past-tense verbs. The presentation of the language isn't traditional either. The explanations are written for veterinarians, not grammarians, so you won't find terms such as "pluperfect" here. Purists may cringe, but the goals are clarity and ease of understanding, not purity.

A note about the dictionary: It, too, is presented in a nontraditional way. Most Spanish–English dictionaries are divided into two parts, one from English to Spanish, and the other from Spanish to English. That has always seemed awkward to us, so we've placed all the language in one section so that you can look up words rapidly. The Spanish letters *ch*, *ll*, and *rr*, which are alphabetized separately in Spanish dictionaries, are not separate in this one; instead, they are included according to the English alphabet. As with the grammar, practicality is our goal, not following the customs of language professionals.

Although you should try for good pronunciation, accurate vocabulary, and clear sentences, you should also know the Great Teachers' Secret: Comprehensible communication can be carried out in imperfect Spanish. If you slip up and say *el anemia* instead of *la anemia*, your client won't stalk out in a huff.

Moreover, the client will get the idea that you're talking about anemia, a subject likely to be of such interest that the *el/la* question is forgotten and probably not even noticed. Really rotten pronunciation does block comprehension, but mildly bad pronunciation does not. We are not encouraging you to be lazy or offhanded in your studies; we are saying that you should relax and speak up. Bad Spanish is better than no Spanish at all. Good Spanish is both useful and a pleasure.

There are many Spanish-speaking countries, each with its own variations in the language. Colombians speak slightly differently from Peruvians; Cubans speak differently from Spaniards. In your area of the United States, listen for dialectical differences in both pronunciation and vocabulary. For instance, there may be many Dominicans in your city, and their Caribbean Spanish is quite different from, say, the Andean Spanish of Bolivia. When writing this book, we tended to favor Mexican Spanish for the simple reason that there are so many people of Mexican background in the United States. However, the language presented here should be comprehensible to all Spanish speakers.

If you work more with large animals than small ones, you should obtain the companion volume to this one, *Spanish for Animal Scientists and Food Animal Producers*.

Meanwhile, *¡buena suerte y bienvenidos al* Español para Veterinarios! (Good luck and welcome to *Spanish for Veterinarians*!)

Acknowledgments

The creation of the course "Spanish for Veterinarians" began as part of an effort to internationalize the curriculum at Washington State University's College of Veterinary Medicine. This effort was carried out with the generous collaboration of the USDA's International Animal Plant Health Inspection Service, the Food and Agriculture Organization, Boehringer Ingelheim Animal Health, Mallinckrodt Veterinary, Pharmacia, and Upjohn. The many-faceted project was designed and directed by Dr. Guy Palmer and Dr. Michael Goe. The authors express their gratitude to Professors Palmer and Goe for allowing us to participate in this exciting endeavor, and we also express our thanks to the forward-thinking organizations that supported it.

The students who suffered through our first, tentative versions of the course deserve special recognition for their patience and dedication. Much of the content of this book was determined by their questions and guidance. It was a true delight to teach WSU's fine veterinary students.

We also thank these local veterinarians who volunteered their help for the first edition: Dr. Victoria Kendall of Cedar Veterinary Hospital, Moscow, Idaho; Dr. Linda Robinette of Alpine Animal Hospital, Pullman, Washington; and Dr. David Roen of Clarkston, Washington.

For this second edition, we are grateful for the help and encouragement of: Banfield Pet Hospital, Fort Worth, Texas; Dr. Russell Johnston of Chisholm Ridge Pet Hospital, Saginaw, Texas; Dr. Steve Lozzi, Wedgwood Animal Hospital, Fort Worth, Texas; Mercedes Place Animal Hospital, Benbrook, Texas; and Dr. Craig Verwers, Ridglea West Animal Hospital, Fort Worth, Texas.

Spanish for Veterinarians

A Practical Introduction

Second Edition

CHAPTER 1

Getting Started

Pronunciation of Spanish

English speakers can breathe a sigh of relief: Unlike English, Spanish is logical and systematic in its pronunciation. There is only one silent letter, and all the other letters have only one major pronunciation. English speakers should focus first on the vowels.

Vowels

a as in f<u>a</u>ther, <u>o</u>tter, m<u>o</u>dern
e as in <u>a</u>ble, <u>ei</u>ght, p<u>ai</u>nt
i as in <u>ea</u>sy, <u>ea</u>t, mach<u>i</u>ne
o as in <u>o</u>ld, r<u>o</u>pe, <u>oa</u>ts
u as in l<u>oo</u>p, m<u>oo</u>, d<u>u</u>de

Now try out the following words, saying them out loud and paying great attention to the vowels (don't worry about anything else yet):

abomaso
abdomen
epidemia
enterovirus
insecto
inseminar
ovario
oviducto
uremia
ubre

Generally speaking, the vowels are more important in the Spanish language than in the English language, so you should practice them as much as possible.

Consonants

Consonants in Spanish are similar to those in English, with these exceptions:

- *d* is soft; it's similar to <u>th</u>ese. When the *d* occurs between two vowels, it might even disappear in rapid speech; *hablado* can become *hablao* in some varieties of Spanish. Some practice words are: *edad, nutrido,* and *ganado.*

- *h* is silent. No matter how tempting it is, it is never pronounced. Some practice words are: *heno, hormona, harina,* and *ahora.*

- *j* is pronounced like the English <u>h</u>appy. Some practice words are: *jinete, conejo,* and *paja.*

- *ll* is pronounced like the English <u>y</u>ahoo. But in some dialects, such as those in Argentina, it's pronounced like <u>j</u>ello. Some practice words are: *caballo, llano,* and *gallina.*

- *ñ* is pronounced like the English ca<u>ny</u>on; the word in Spanish is *cañón.* Some practice words are: *año, ordeño,* and *rapiña.*

- *qu* is pronounced like the English <u>k</u>ick, not <u>qu</u>ick; it doesn't have the *w* sound as in English. Some practice words are: *que, equino,* and *quiste.*

- *r* inside a word has a little flip of the tongue as in the English words ba<u>tt</u>er, bi<u>tt</u>er, or bu<u>tt</u>er. Practice these words first to loosen up your tongue. Some practice words are: *toro, terapia,* and *ubre.*

- To pronounce *rr* or *r* at the beginning of a word, you must first practice purring like a cat or making a sound like a car revving up. The sound should be in your tongue (flapping like a flag in the wind) and not in your throat (no hacking please). As before, you should loosen your tongue. Some practice words are: *perro, rabia, rumiante,* and *forraje.* NOTE: The tongue muscles you use to make this revving sound are not commonly used in English, so yours are probably not accustomed to making this sound. If you notice that the sides of your tongue are a little sore, that means you're practicing this sound properly, and those muscles are getting stronger.

- *v* is pronounced like the English <u>b</u>ed. A common spelling mistake among native Spanish speakers is to substitute *b* for *v* and vice versa. Some practice words are: *vaca, virus,* and *veterinario.*

- *x* is usually pronounced as it is in English; here is *x* in its usual *ks* form: *toxina, examen, sexo,* and *ixodicida.* But in certain words taken from the indigenous groups, *x* is more like the Spanish *j.* A practice word is *México.*

- *z* is pronounced like *s* in Latin America, but it is pronounced like *th* by many Spaniards. Some practice words to try both ways are: *pezuña*, *lechuza*, and *enzima*.

- *c* and *g* can be hard or soft, depending on what follows. *C* is hard like *k* when it is followed by *a*, *o*, or *u*. Some practice words are: *caballo*, *cola*, and *curar*. But it is soft like *s* when it is followed by *i* or *e*. Some practice words are: *ciencia* and *cebra*. Similarly, *g* is pronounced like English gargle when it's followed by *a*, *o*, or *u*. Some practice words are: *ganado*, *gallina*, and *gusano*. Followed by *e* or *i*, the *g* becomes softened and is pronounced like English <u>h</u>ello. Some practice words are *gestante*, *ingesta*, and *agitado*.

Which Syllable to Stress?

In Spanish there are three rules for syllable emphasis, that is, which syllable is pronounced stronger than the other parts of the word.

1. If a word ends in a vowel, *s*, or *n*, then the stress is on the next-to-last syllable. Some examples are: *s<u>a</u>ngre*, *cu<u>e</u>rno*, *ab<u>e</u>ja*, *r<u>a</u>zas*, *cr<u>e</u>cen*, and *d<u>o</u>sis*.

2. If a word ends in a consonant except *s* or *n*, the stress is on the last syllable. Some examples are: *tum<u>o</u>r*, *morbosid<u>a</u>d*, *est<u>a</u>r*, and *rur<u>a</u>l*.

3. If a word doesn't follow rule 1 or rule 2, then there's a written accent mark. Some examples are: *pájaro*, *gládula*, *ácaro*, *trébol*, and *mamífero*.

Nouns and Plurals

Nouns are things or objects; in English, you can spot a noun because it can have the article "the" in front of it: the house, the barn, or the doctor. In Spanish, all nouns have gender; they are either masculine or feminine.

Feminine nouns often end in *a*, and their version of the article "the" is *la*: *la vaca*, *la oveja*, *la pata*, *la cola*, and *la pipa*.

Masculine nouns often end in *o*, and their version of the article "the" is *el*: *el caballo*, *el perro*, *el calcio*, and *el rebaño*. There are, however, exceptions, such as *la mano* or *la radio*.

Words that end in *-itis*, *-osis*, *-ción*, *-dad*, *-tad*, *-tud*, *-ie*, or *-umbre* are usually feminine. Some examples are *la mastitis*, *la pediculosis*, *la inyección*, *la obesidad*, *la dificultad*, *la multitud*, *la serie*, and *la certidumbre*.

The Spanish language also absorbed many Greek words. In Greek, a word ending in *a* is masculine. Some examples are: *el síntoma, el edema, el sistema, el mapa, el problema, el programa, el linfoma, el enfisema,* and *el tema.* Notice that most, though not all, of these words end in *-ema.*

Beyond these guidelines, you simply have to learn the gender of the noun when you learn the noun. As you study vocabulary, always learn the word with its article *el* or *la.* Notice, for example, that the following words both end in *e,* but they differ in gender: *la sangre* and *el forraje.*

When it comes to people and animals, there often are pairs of words showing the actual gender of the person or animal.

> *la especialista, el especialista; la veterinaria, el veterinario; la dueña, el dueño; la gata, el gato; la coneja, el conejo; la perra, el perro*

Articles and Plurals

As was previously discussed, the definite article "the" in English is equivalent to *la* or *el* in Spanish. The indefinite article "a" or "an" in English is equivalent to *una* (feminine) or *un* (masculine) in Spanish:

> *la pluma* (**the feather**)   *una pluma* (**a feather**)
> *el gusano* (**the worm**)   *un gusano* (**a worm**)

If the word ends in a vowel, just add *s* to make the nouns and articles plural because both have to match in both gender and number:

> *las plumas* (**the feathers**)   *unas plumas* (**some feathers**)
> *los gusanos* (**the worms**)   *unos gusanos* (**some worms**)

If the word ends in a consonant, add *es* to make the noun and article plural:

> *el tumor* (**the tumor**)   *los tumores* (**the tumors**)
> *la edad* (**the age**)   *las edades* (**the ages**)

Names of Animals

EXERCISE 1-1

Practice saying the following vocabulary out loud. To hear these as pronounced by native speakers, go to www.span.tcu.edu/vet_spanish. You can download the pronunciation exercises, so that you can practice speaking Spanish. Also, if you have Spanish-speaking friends or clients, there's nothing like practicing with a real live human being.

Los animales domésticos (Domestic animals).

English	Male	Female	Offspring	Collective form, such as herd or flock
Cattle	*El toro*	*La vaca*	*La ternera* *El ternero*	*El ganado*
Horses	*El caballo*	*La yegua*	*La potranca* *El potro*	*La manada*
Chickens	*El gallo*	*La gallina*	*La pollita* *El pollito*	*La parvada*
Dogs	*El perro*	*La perra*	*La cachorra* *El cachorro*	*La jauría*
Cats	*El gato*	*La gata*	*La gatita* *El gatito*	*Los gatos*
Goats	*El macho cabrío* *La cabra macho*	*La cabra*	*La cabrita* *El cabrito*	*El rebaño*
Sheep	*El carnero*	*La oveja*	*La cordera* *El cordero*	*El rebaño*
Swine	*El cerdo*	*La cerda*	*La lechona* *El lechón*	*La piara*
Ducks	*El pato*	*La pata*	*La patita* *El patito*	*La bandada*
Rabbits	*El conejo*	*La coneja*	*La conejita* *El conejito*	*Los conejos*

EXERCISE 1-2

Now write the plural form of each vocabulary word from Exercise 1-1. For example: *el toro, los toros; la vaca, las vacas,* and so on. As you write out the word, say it out loud. When you're done, check your answers against the Answer Key at the end of the book.

EXERCISE 1-3

Write each vocabulary word using the indefinite article instead of the definite one. For example: *el toro, un toro.*

EXERCISE 1-4

Pronounce the following vocabulary words out loud, then practice them again with the help of www.span.tcu.edu/vet_spanish.

Some Wild Animals *(Algunos animales salvajes)*

Antelope	**(el antípole)**
Bear	**(el oso)**
Camel	**(el camello)**
Crocodile	**(el cocodrilo)**
Deer	**(el venado, el ciervo)**
Elephant	**(el elefante)**
Fish	**(el pez)**
Fox	**(el zorro)**
Giraffe	**(la jirafa)**
Hippopotamus	**(el hipopótamo)**
Lion	**(el león)**
Llama	**(la llama)**
Monkey	**(el mono)**
Ostrich	**(el avestruz)**
Rhinoceros	**(el rinoceronte)**
Shark	**(el tiburón)**
Snake	**(la serpiente, la culebra)**
Tiger	**(el tigre)**
Whale	**(la ballena)**
Zebra	**(la cebra)**

EXERCISE 1-5

Now write the plurals of the vocabulary in Exercise 1-4. Be sure to say the words out loud as you write them. For example: *el oso, los osos.*

EXERCISE 1-6

Write each vocabulary word in Exercise 1-4 with the indefinite article instead of the definite one. For example: *el oso, un oso.*

EXERCISE 1-7

These words may look like English words, but they're not. Pronounce them as best as you can using the rules provided in this chapter.

rancho
elefante
teléfono
animal
cliente
medicina
vitamina
biología
análisis
diarrea
virus
pie
mastitis
pus
natural
color
tumor
dieta

CULTURAL NOTE

Surnames

Names in Hispanic societies include both the patronymic (the father's last name) and the matronymic (the mother's last name). Here's an example: Juan González Aranda. González is Juan's father's last name, and Aranda is his mother's maiden name. Juan can sign his name either Juan González Aranda or simply Juan González. Let's imagine that Juan marries María Hernández Luna. Their adorable daughter Elena takes both parents' patronymic names, so she is Elena González Hernández. She can sign her name Elena González Hernández or simply Elena González.

A married woman can, if she wants, add her husband's name by putting *de* with his last name after her own. For example, María could be María Hernández Luna de González. Or she can remain María Hernández Luna. Or she can be María Hernández de

González. But she isn't María González unless she moves to the United States.

If you have Spanish-language check-in forms, you can show respect for this naming system by leaving space for *apellido(s)* (last name[s]). If your client fills in the blank with, say, García Rodríguez, the form should be filed under "G" for García. García, by the way, is the most common last name in Spanish-speaking cultures; it is like Smith in English-speaking ones. One way to get an idea of the size of the Hispanic community in your town is to count the number of Garcías in the phone book.

The Body and How to Describe It

Adjectives

An adjective is a word that describes a noun. It shares the same gender and number as the noun it describes. In Spanish, the adjective usually follows the noun, rather than preceding it as in English.

For example, *la pata* (the paw) is a singular, feminine noun. So its adjective must be singular and feminine, too; *una pata inflamada* (an inflamed paw), as in *mi gato tiene una pata inflamada* (my cat has an inflamed paw).

la pata hinchada (**the swollen paw**)
una pata lastimada (**an injured paw**)
la pata blanca (**the white paw**)

If the noun becomes plural, so, too, does its adjective:

unas patas inflamadas (**some inflamed paws**)
las patas hinchadas (**the swollen paws**)
unas patas lastimadas (**some injured paws**)
las patas blancas (**the white paws**)

Here's another example: *el ojo* (the eye) is a singular, masculine noun. So its adjective must be singular and masculine, too; *un ojo inflamado* (an inflamed eye), as in *la vaca tiene un ojo inflamado* (the cow has an inflamed eye).

un ojo lloroso (**a watery, teary eye**)
el ojo ciego (**the blind eye**)
el ojo pardo (**the brown eye**)

If the noun becomes plural, so, too, does its adjective:

unos ojos inflamados (**some inflamed eyes**)
unos ojos llorosos (**some watery, teary eyes**)

los ojos ciegos (**the blind eyes**)
los ojos pardos (**the brown eyes**)

Forming plurals is the same for adjectives as for nouns. If the word ends in a vowel, just add *s*. If it ends in a consonant, add *es*.

el ojo azul (**the blue eye**)
los ojos azules (**the blue eyes**)

Naturally, all rules need exceptions. In this case, the exception has to do with numbers: They go before the noun, not after it, and they don't change their endings for number or gender.

cuatro patas (**four feet**) Contrast this with *patas blancas* (**white feet**)
ocho vacas (**eight cows**).

Words that indicate amount, like other adjectives, do change, but they are placed before the noun, like numbers.

muchos caballos (**many horses, a lot of horses**)
pocas llamas (**few llamas, not many llamas**)
mucho trabajo (**a lot of work**)

CULTURAL NOTE

To indicate a castrated animal, use either the adjective *capado* (often used for male animals) or *castrada* (often used for female animals). Examples:

barrow   *el cerdo capado*
spayed cat   *la gata castrada, el gato capado*
wether   *el carnero capado*
gelding   *el caballo capado*

EXERCISE 2-1

Apply the adjective to the nouns following it. Example: *hinchado*

la pierna, la pierna hinchada
las piernas, las piernas hinchadas

1. (blanco)
   el caballo
   la gata
   los cerdos

2. (lastimado)
   la pata
   las piernas
   los pies
   el ojo

3. (enfermo)
   el perro
   las cebras
   los cabritos
   la oveja

4. (cinco)
   las pulgas
   los tumores
   los días

5. (mucho)
   los animales
   las infecciones
   la sangre
   el olor

6. (sanguinolenta)
   la orina
   las heces
   el moco
   el vómito

7. (posible)
   el diagnóstico
   los problemas
   la solución
   las terapias

8. (respiratorio)
   una enfermedad
   un ruido
   los problemas
   los exámenes

EXERCISE 2-2

Substitute the word in parentheses for the underlined word, and make any necessary changes in the adjective. Example: <u>la respiración</u> normal (las pruebas) should be *las pruebas normales*.

1. <u>el gato</u> anémico (la gata)
2. <u>el vómito</u> frecuente (las convulsiones)
3. <u>la vaca</u> letárgica (el cerdo)
4. <u>el tumor</u> pequeño (los quistes)
5. <u>el vértigo</u> repentino (las fiebres)
6. <u>la pata</u> lastimada (las costillas)
7. <u>la orina</u> dificultosa (el parto)
8. poco <u>apetito</u> (la energía)
9. <u>la perra</u> capada (los perros)
10. <u>los problemas</u> respiratorios (la dificultad)

External Body Parts (*Las partes corporales externas*)────

With the help of www.span.tcu.edu/vet_spanish, practice the pronunciation of these body parts.

el ala (**wing**)
la almohadilla (**paw pad**)
la boca, la faringe (**mouth**)
la cabeza (**head**)
la caña (**shank**)
la cola (**tail**)
la coronilla (**poll**)
la cresta (**comb**)
la cruz (**withers**)
la cuartilla (**pastern**)
el cuello (**neck**)
el cuerno (**horn**)
el dedo (**toe**)
el escroto (**scrotum**)
el flanco (**flank**)
la grupa (**rump**)
el hocico (**muzzle**)
el hombro (**shoulder**)
la joroba (**hump**)
el menudillo (**fetlock**)

el ojo (**eye**)
el ollar (**nostril**)
la oreja (**ear**)
la pata (**paw**)
el pelo (**hair, fur, pelt**)
el pene (**penis**)
la pezuña, el casco (**hoof**)
el pico (**beak**)
el pie (**foot**)
la piel (**skin, hide**)
la pierna (**leg**)
la pluma (**feather**)
la rodilla (**knee**)
el talón (**heel**)
el tarso, el corvejón (**hock**)
el testículo (**testicle**)
la teta (**teat**)
el tórax (**thorax**)
la ubre (**udder**)
la uña (**nail**)

Internal Organs (*Los órganos internos*)

Practice the pronunciation of these internal organs.

el abdomen (**abdomen**)
el ano (**anus**)
el buche (**crop, craw**)
el cerebro, el encéfalo (**brain**)
el colon (**colon**)
el corazón (**heart**)
el esófago (**esophagus**)
el estómago (**stomach**)
el garguero (**gullet**)
la glándula (**gland**)
el hígado (**liver**)
el intestino, las tripas (**intestines**)
la molleja (**gizzard**)
el nervio (**nerve**)

el ovario (**ovary**)
la placenta (**placenta**)
el pulmón (**lung**)
el recto (**rectum**)
el riñón (**kidney**)
el rumen (**rumen**)
la tráquea (**trachea**)
el útero (**uterus**)
la vagina (**vagina**)
la vejiga *or* la vesícula urinaria (**urinary bladder**)
la vena yugular (**jugular vein**)
la vesícula biliar (**gallbladder**)
la vulva (**vulva**)

EXERCISE 2-3

Using the dictionary at the back of the book, find the Spanish equivalent of the English word in parentheses. Make sure that it corresponds in gender and number with the noun it describes. Example: *los músculos* (weak) should be *los músculos débiles.*

1. el abdomen (distended)
2. los ojos (watery)
3. la almohadilla (infected)
4. el corazón (irregular)
5. la vulva (bloody)
6. la boca (dry)
7. los perros (newborn)
8. los pulmones (congested)
9. el ano (impacted)
10. las tripas (equine)

Write the correct definite article for the noun.

1. _____ rodillas
2. _____ hocico
3. _____ cabra
4. _____ problema
5. _____ sangre
6. _____ mastitis
7. _____ fiebre
8. _____ cuernos
9. _____ cruz
10. _____ ubre
11. _____ gatas
12. _____ enfermedades
13. _____ osos
14. _____ pez

15. _____ plumas
16. _____ sorgo .
17. _____ vitaminas
18. _____ suplementos
19. _____ tórax
20. _____ síntoma
21. _____ moquillo
22. _____ diarrea
23. _____ llamas
24. _____ animal
25. _____ uña
26. _____ infecciones
27. _____ pata
28. _____ ojo

How Can I Learn All This Vocabulary?

The most efficient way to learn vocabulary is through the old-fashioned technique of flash cards. Cut up some paper into squares about the size of your driver's license. Write the Spanish word on one side (don't forget the *el* or *la*) and the English equivalent on the other side. Simply preparing the cards is a good study exercise in itself. If you have an exclusively large animal practice, you won't need to learn the vocabulary for small animals, and vice versa.

Now practice. First, look at the Spanish word and make your guess about the English word. If you get it right, put it in one pile. If you get it wrong, put it in another. At the end, redo the words in the pile of the words that you missed until you get them right. And then reverse the process. Look at the English word and guess the Spanish word, sorting your answers into two piles as you did before.

Practice a few minutes each day, including both Spanish to English and English to Spanish. Don't spend hours at it, or you'll bore yourself and make it harder to study. But keep your cards handy. During TV commercials, while you're waiting in line at the bank, while you're sitting in the doctor's waiting room—these are all good moments to pull out your flash cards and practice.

Everyone has one or two words that they never learn, no matter how often they practice. Who knows why? It must be some trick of the human brain, or maybe it's Greek hubris. Aren't there a few words in English that you never spell correctly, no matter how many times you look them up? In any case, don't beat yourself up if you miss the Spanish word for "bladder" every single time.

Keep old flash cards in a shoe box so that you can refresh your memory from time to time. Studies show that lots of repetition, spread out over a period of time, produces the best long-term learning.

CULTURAL NOTE

Greeting Clients

Personal interaction is more important in Spanish-speaking cultures than in English-speaking ones. The impersonality of business behaviors in the United States might seem professional to Anglos and others who are accustomed to this impersonal style, but it can seem cold and unwelcoming to Hispanics and others who are not accustomed to it. For this reason, it is appropriate to greet your Spanish-speaking clients a little more thoroughly than your English-speaking ones would expect.

- Shake hands at the the beginning *and* the end of the consultation. Handshakes in the Hispanic world don't involve a lot of squeezing; they're more hand touches than grasps. Don't pump vigorously; just a gentle, brief up-and-down motion is enough. If there are several people, shake hands with everyone in the group.
- As you shake hands, introduce yourself and use a variety of the polite phrases given here. The important thing is to acknowledge the presence of each person with a handshake and a spoken phrase.
- Now the consultation can begin. Stand a little closer to the client than you would with an English-speaking client. Normal personal space is much closer in Hispanic culture than in Anglo culture, so you may feel a little uncomfortable, but it will feel right to your client. Look the clients in the face, but don't stare into their eyes. Nonprofessional people may keep their eyes lowered in front of

you because in Hispanic cultures, it is considered proper to lower one's eyes in front of authorities, such as medical personnel, teachers, and police.

- At the end of the consultation, shake hands again and use one of the provided phrases again.

Some Polite Greetings and Phrases

Soy doctor Smith. [**I am doctor** *(male)* **Smith.**] *Soy doctora Smith.*
   [**I am doctor** *(female)* **Smith.**]
Mucho gusto. [**Pleased to meet you.**]
Encantado. [**Delighted,** *(male)*.] *Encantada.* [**Delighted,** *(female)*.]
Buenos días. [**Good morning.**]
Buenas tardes. [**Good afternoon; Good evening.**]
NOTE: *Hola* (Hi) is too informal for a doctor–client conversation.
¿Cómo está usted, señor García? [**How are you, Mr. García?**]
Estoy bien, gracias. [**I'm fine, thank you.**]
Bueno. Vamos a ver. [**OK. Let's see now.**]
Nos vemos la próxima semana. [**See you next week.**]
Vuelva usted en dos semanas. [**Come back in two weeks.**]
Gracias por su visita. [**Thank you for your visit.**]
Hasta luego. [**Until then; until soon.**]

CHAPTER 3

Verbs: Where the Action Is

Regular Verbs

Verbs are the words that indicate actions. Put a verb together with a dog, and the dog can run, sleep, sit, beg, and bark. Verbs carry most of the meaning in a sentence, so it's important to understand them and be able to use them with ease.

All the verbs in the Spanish language have an infinitive form and end in *-ar*, *-er*, or *-ir*. The infinitive form translates as "to": *tratar* (to treat), *correr* (to run), and *vivir* (to live).

Spanish verbs change according to who is doing the action. You can see this in English, too: I go, she goes, or we go. The form the verb takes specifically indicates who is carrying out the action, so that the noun or pronoun itself is often unnecessary in Spanish.

Yo (I) is indicated in the verb by breaking off the infinitive ending (*-ar*, *-er*, *-ir*) and adding *-o*:

Tratar	*yo trato* [**I treat**]
Correr	*yo corro* [**I run**]
Vivir	*yo vivo* [**I live**]

Nosotros (we) is indicated in the verb by breaking off the infinitive ending and adding *-amos*, *-emos*, or *-imos*.

Tratar	*tratamos* [**we treat**]
Correr	*corremos* [**we run**]
Vivir	*vivimos* [**we live**]

Ella, *él*, and *usted* (she, he, and you [formal]) are indicated in the verb by breaking off the infinitive ending and adding *-a* or *-e*.

Tratar	*trata* [she treats, he treats, you treat]
Correr	*corre* [she runs, he runs, you run]
Vivir	*vive* [she lives, he lives, you live]

Ellas, ellos, ustedes (they, you all or you guys) are indicated in the verb by breaking off the infinitive ending and adding *-an* or *-en*:

Tratar	*tratan* [they treat, you all or you guys treat]
Correr	*corren* [they run, you all run]
Vivir	*viven* [they live, you all live]

Tú is the form of you that is used only to address good friends, children, animals, or God. You wouldn't use this form with professional clients; with them, you'll use *usted*. *Tú* is indicated in the verb by breaking off the infinitive ending and adding *-as* or *-es*.

Tratar	*tratas* [you treat]
Correr	*corres* [you run]
Vivir	*vives* [you live]

Here is *tratar* again, this time with all its forms:

trato [I treat]
tratamos [we treat]
tratas [you (informal) treat]
trata [she treats, he treats, you (formal) treat]
tratan [they treat, you all treat]

It's customary to run a verb through its paces by putting it in a chart like this, with the singulars in one column and the plurals in another.

yo trato	*nosotros tratamos*
tú tratas	
él, ella, usted trata	*ellos, ellas, ustedes tratan*

CULTURAL NOTE

In Spanish there's no "it treats." All things are either masculine or feminine in Spanish, so the equivalent in Spanish is "he treats" or "she treats." For example, when you describe the use of a pill because it is feminine *(la pastilla)* you'll say, "she treats inflammation." Looking at an inner ear because it is masculine *(el oído)*, you'll say "he is infected."

EXERCISE 3-1

Write out the conjugations of these verbs. You may omit the *tú* form if you like.

1. vendar (**to bandage**)
2. revisar (**to check over**)
3. inocular (**to inoculate**)
4. comprender (**to understand**)
5. deber (**to ought to, should**)
6. creer (**to believe, to think**)
7. añadir (**to add**)
8. recibir (**to receive**)
9. sufrir (**to suffer**)
10. ordeñar (**to milk**)

EXERCISE 3-2

With many of the verbs you'll use in your veterinary practice, you only need to know two forms because you will not be using them to discuss your own or your client's actions. For example, for *rascar* (to scratch an itch), you only need to practice *rasca* (e.g., the dog scratches) and *rascan* (e.g., the dogs scratch). For each of the following verbs, write the forms that match the subjects indicated.

1. parir (**to give birth**), the sow, the sows
2. lamer (**to lick**), the cat, the cats
3. ocurrir (**to occur**), the problem, the problems
4. toser (**to cough**), the puppy, the puppies
5. respirar (**to breathe**), the mare, the mares
6. jadear (**to pant**), the dog, the dogs
7. comer (**to eat**), the parrot, the parrots
8. padecer de (**to suffer from**), the ewe, the ewes
9. parecer (**to seem**), the wound, the wounds
10. cojear (**to limp**), the llama, the llamas

EXERCISE 3-3

Fill in the blanks with the proper form of the verb. Example: *Yo __examino__ (examinar) los animales con cuidado.*

1. El caballo _____ (padecer) de cólico.
2. La vaca _____ (toser) con dolor.
3. El corazón _____ (latir) muy rápido.

4. Nosotros _____ (revisar) los síntomas.
5. ¿Usted _____ (vendar) la herida diariamente?
6. Yo _____ (creer) que necesita vitaminas.
7. Las plumas _____ (parecer) pálidas.
8. Ustedes _____ (limpiar) la jaula regularmente.
9. El medicamento _____ (deber) curar el problema.
10. Las llamas _____ (beber) y _____
    (comer) normalmente.

Weak-Kneed Verbs

When they're surrounded by strong, aggressive consonants, some vowels fall apart when the pronounced stress falls on them. For example, *e* has a habit of breaking down into *ie* or *i*, and *o* commonly breaks down into *ue*. Here is an example:

Tender (ie) [**to tend**]

yo tiendo	*nosotros tendemos*
tú tiendes	
él, ella, usted tiende	*ellos, ellas, ustedes tienden*

Why did the *e* break down in *tiende* but not in *tendemos*? Because the stress in *tendemos* falls not on the *e* in the vulnerable position between two aggressive consonants but on the ending *-emos*, which has gentler consonants. Here's another example; watch where it falls apart and where it doesn't:

Dormir (ue) [**to sleep**]

yo duermo	*nosotros dormimos*
tú duermes	
él, ella, usted duerme	*ellos, ellas, ustedes duermen*

The change occurs in all forms except the *nosotros* form. In the dictionary, you'll see the change in parentheses after the infinitive: *dormir* (ue). That way, you'll know that the verb has a vulnerable vowel.

EXERCISE 3-4

On a sheet of scratch paper, conjugate the following weak-kneed verbs. The vulnerable vowel is underlined.

1. recom<u>e</u>ndar (ie) **(to recommend)**
2. qu<u>e</u>rer (ie) **(to want)**
3. sug<u>e</u>rir (ie) **(to suggest)**
4. p<u>e</u>rder (ie) **(to lose)**
5. t<u>e</u>mblar (ie) **(to tremble)**
6. pr<u>o</u>bar (ue) **(to prove)**
7. p<u>o</u>der (ue) **(to be able, can, may)**
8. v<u>o</u>lver (ue) **(to return)**
9. s<u>e</u>guir (i) **(to follow, to keep on)**
10. p<u>e</u>dir (i) **(to ask for, to request)**

EXERCISE 3-5

Conjugate these verbs only in the he or she and they forms.

1. c<u>o</u>star (ue) **(to cost)**
2. v<u>o</u>lar (ue) **(to fly)**
3. m<u>o</u>rder (ue) **(to bite)**
4. prev<u>e</u>nir (ie) **(to prevent)**
5. <u>o</u>ler (ue) **(to smell,** in the sense of having odor) Note: add "h" in front of the conjugated forms.
6. m<u>o</u>strar (ue) **(to show signs of)**

EXERCISE 3-6

Fill in the blanks with the proper form of the verb in parentheses.

1. El gato _____ (temblar) mucho debido a la fiebre.
2. Los síntomas _____ (volver) después de terminar el tratamiento.
3. Yo _____ (recomendar) unos suplementos de vitaminas.
4. Mi esposa y yo _____ (querer) lo mejor para "Spot."
5. ¿ _____ (poder) usted volver en tres días?
6. Los resultados _____ (probar) que la vaca tiene anaplasmosis.
7. El antibiótico _____ (costar) mucho pero es el mejor remedio para este problema.

8. Frecuentemente, la infección _____ (seguir) después de una herida en la piel.

9. Si los animales _____ (perder) peso rapidamente, indica la presencia de una enfermedad.

10. Nosostros _____ (recomendar) una serie de inyecciones.

11. El señor Ramírez _____ (pedir) una revisión de su ganado para el próximo jueves.

How Should I Study Verbs?

There are two things to study about verbs: (1) the meaning of the infinitive and (2) the conjugation. Prepare flash cards as described previously for the meanings. If the verb is weak-kneed, don't forget to indicate that; example: *perder* (ie).

Learning conjugations is done by writing. On scratch paper, write out the conjugation of the verbs you've learned in this chapter. Do about five verbs once a day for two weeks. Don't just look at the verb and conjugate it mentally; you have to include physical movement (that is, your arm moving over the paper) to engrave something in your memory. The people who study learning say that the more physical senses you include, the better you'll learn. So if you say the words out loud as you write them, you're including several physical senses (touch, hearing, and sight) and you'll learn faster and better.

More than 70 percent of all Spanish verbs are regular *-ar* ones, conjugated like *tratar*. So, if you know these endings, you'll have most of the verbs mastered.

Writing out verb conjugations is not exciting, but it is a good study method. As in the case of flash cards, don't do it too long or you'll give up. But what else do you have to do during TV commercials? And think how much fun it'll be to answer the phone and say, "Oh, I was just sitting here conjugating."

Irregular Verbs

Four Essential Irregular Verbs: *tener*, *estar*, *ser*, and *ir*_____

It would be too easy if all Spanish verbs followed the regular patterns you learned in the previous chapter, but they do not. There are irregular verbs, too. Four of them are so common that they appear in every conversation. They are *tener* (to have), *ser* (to be), *estar* (to be, to become), and *ir* (to go).

Here are the conjugations of these essential verbs:

tener

tengo (**I have**)	*tenemos* (**we have**)
tienes (**you [informal] have**)	
tiene (**he or she has; you [formal] have**)	*tienen* (**they, you all have**)

estar

estoy (**I am**)	*estamos* (**we are**)
estás (**you [informal] are**)	
está (**he or she is; you [formal] are**)	*están* (**they, you all are**)

ser

soy (**I am**)	*somos* (**we are**)
eres (**you [informal] are**)	
es (**he or she is; you [formal] are**)	*son* (**they, you all are**)

ir

voy **(I go)**	*vamos* **(we go)**
vas **(you [informal] go)**	
va **(he or she goes; you [formal] go)**	*van* **(they, you all go)**

Tener [to have]

Tener is used with nouns, such as the following list demonstrates. With *tener* the noun doesn't always have to have an article.

¿Qué tiene el animal? **[What's the matter with the animal? (Literally, what does the animal have?)]**

El animal tiene . . . **[The animal has . . .]**

garrapatas **(ticks)**	*parvovirus* **(parvovirus)**
gusanos **(worms)**	*fiebre* **(fever)**
mastitis **(mastitis)**	*laminitis* **(laminitis)**
heces secas **(dry droppings)**	*diarrea* **(diarrhea)**
cólico **(colic)**	*leucemia* **(leukemia)**
vómito **(vomiting)**	*sarna* **(mange)**
neumonía **(pneumonia)**	*septicemia* **(blood poisoning)**
tos **(a cough)**	*hematuria* **(hematuria)**
letargo **(lethargy)**	*anemia* **(anemia)**
artritis **(arthritis)**	*ácaros* **(mites)**
un quiste **(a cyst)**	*hidropesía* **(dropsy)**
constipación **(constipation)**	*arritmia* **(arrythmia)**
el moquillo **(distemper)**	*gangrena* **(gangrene)**
erisipela **(erysipelas)**	*hemofilia* **(hemophilia)**
pulso normal **(normal pulse)**	*parásitos* **(parasites)**
temblores **(shivering)**	*convulsiones* **(seizures)**
hemorragias **(hemorrhages)**	*dolor* **(pain)**

Once you know how to conjugate *tener*, you can also conjugate other verbs that contain *tener*. These forms of *tener* also use the same forms.

Mantener	**(to maintain, to keep)**
Contener	**(to contain)**
Retener	**(to retain)**
Detener	**(to detain)**
Obtener	**(to obtain)**
Sostener	**(to sustain, to hold still)**

Estar [to be]

Estar is used with adjectives, such as the list of following conditions shows. Remember that the adjective reflects the gender and number of the thing it refers to.

La vaca está . . . [**The cow is . . .**]

gestante (**pregnant**)	*mal* (**bad off, poorly**)
bien (**fine**)	*enferma* (**sick**)
ciega (**blind**)	*atáxica* (**atactic**)
moribunda (**dying**)	*grave* (**gravely ill**)
fértile, fecunda (**fertile**)	*infétil, estéril* (**sterile**)
congestionada (**congested**)	*débil* (**weak**)

El ojo está . . . [**The eye is . . .**]

lloroso (**watery**)	*inflamado* (**inflamed**)
hundido (**sunken**)	*turbio* (**cloudy**)
irritado (**irritated**)	*mejor* (**better**)
peor (**worse**)	*amarillento* (**yellowish**)

Las mucosas están . . . [**The mucous membranes are . . .**]

congestionadas (**congested**)	*pálidas* (**pale, whitish**)
normales (**normal**)	*secas* (**dry**)
ictéricas (**icteric**)	*cianóticas* (**cyanotic**)

La orina está . . . [**The urine is . . .**]

concentrada (**concentrated**)	*sanguinolenta* (**bloody**)
fétida (**fetid**)	*turbia* (**cloudy**)

El loro está . . . [**The parrot is . . .**]

pálido (**pallid, pale**)	*letárgico* (**lethargic**)
peor (**worse**)	*agitado* (**agitated**)
flaco (**thin, too thin**)	*lastimado* (**injured**)

Ser [to be]

Ser is used for identity, profession, personality, and physical characteristics that one is born with. It can be used with adjectives or nouns.

El señor Valdés es . . . [**Mr. Valdés is . . .**]

veterinario (**a veterinarian**)	*argentino* (**Argentine**)
alto (**tall**)	*moreno* (**brown-haired**)
simpático (**nice**)	*inteligente* (**intelligent**)

un cliente estimado (**an esteemed client**)
dueño de la lechería (**owner of the dairy**)

La finca es . . . [**The farm is . . .**]

pequeña (**small**)   *grande* (**big**)
moderna (**modern**)   *productiva* (**productive**)

autosuficiente (**self-sufficient**)
difícil/fácil de encontrar (**hard/easy to find**)

El perro es . . . [**The dog is . . .**]

cruzado (**a mutt**)   *manso* (**tame, docile**)
pardo y negro (**brown and black**)   *juguetón* (**playful**)

la mascota de los García (**the García family's pet**)
pastor alemán (**a German shepherd**)

Mi especialidad profesional es . . . [**My professional specialty is . . .**]

la anatomía patológica (**animal pathology**)
la anestesiología (**anesthesiology**)
el bioanálisis clínico (**clinical bioanalysis**)
la biología celular (**cell biology**)
la ciencia pecuaria (**livestock science**)
la cirugía (**surgery**)
la citopatología o piscícola (**cytology**)
la economía agraria (**agricultural economics**)
la epidemiología (**epidemiology**)
la fisiopatología (**physiopathology**)
la hematología (**hematology**)
la histopatología (**histopathology**)
la inmunología (**immunology**)
la medicina preventiva (**preventive medicine**)
la microbiología (**microbiology**)
la neurología (**neurology**)
la nutrición (**nutrition**)
la odontología (**odontology**)
la oncología veterinaria (**veterinary oncology**)
la optalmología (**ophthalmology**)
la ornitología (**ornithology**)
la parasitología (**parasithology**)
la patología animal (**animal pathology**)
la producción porcina (**swine production**)

la radiología (**radiology**)
la salmonicultura (**salmoniculture**)
la toxicología (**toxicology**)
la virología (**virology**)

Ir [to go]

The verb *ir* is handy. It means "to go" as in "I go to the movies" (*voy al cine*). But it also can be put together with *a* and an infinitive, to make the idea of "going to" (do something). For example, *el veterinario va a examinar el cerdo* means the vet is going to examine the pig.

Ahora, voy a . . . [**Now, I'm going to . . .**]

examinar el ala [**examine the wing**]
vacunar los perritos [**vaccinate the puppies**]
vendar la herida [**bandage the wound**]
tomar la temperatura [**take its temperature**]
recetar una pastillas [**prescribe some pills**]
escuchar el corazón [**listen to its heart**]
consultar con una especialista [**consult with a specialist**]

Este medicamento va a . . . [**This medicine is going to . . .**]

aliviar el dolor (**relieve the pain**)
bajar la fiebre (**lower the fever**)
prevenir una infección (**prevent an infection**)
curar la enfermedad (**cure the illness**)
costar poco/mucho (**cost a little/a lot**)
controlar los signos (**control the symptoms**)
expulsar los parásitos (**get rid of the parasites**)

Other Infinitive Phrases

The *ir a* + infinitive phrase you learned is useful in many situations. And so now, you're probably wondering if there are other infinitive phrases like it. Indeed, there are. Learn these simple infinitive phrases and you will vastly expand your expressive powers.

poder (ue) [**to be able**]
Puedo volver mañana. [**I can return tomorrow.**]

acabar de [**to have just**]
Los resultados de la biopsia acaban de llegar. [**The biopsy results have just arrived.**]

tener que [**to have to**]

Tengo que consultar con los especialistas. [**I have to consult the specialists.**]

volver (ue) *a* [**to do again**]

La cacatúa vuelve a picarse las plumas. [**The cockatoo is picking out its feathers again.**]

deber [**ought to, should**]

Estas gotas deben curar el problema. [**These drops should cure the problem.**]

necesitar [**to need**]

Necesitamos sacar una biopsia. [**We need to take a biopsy.**]

EXERCISE 4-1

Complete the sentence with the appropriate form of *tener, estar, ser,* or *ir*.

1. La orina _____ sanguinolenta.
2. Los cachorros _____ diarrea.
3. El quiste _____ pequeño y no canceroso.
4. Usted _____ que administrar la medicina tres veces el día.
5. La enfermera _____ a inyectar un antibiótico.
6. La tos _____ peor. Creo que _____ neumonía.
7. Las dos cacatúas _____ parásitos.
8. La sarna _____ difícil de tratar.
9. Señora García, su perra _____ débil ahora, pero en unos días, _____ a estar bien.
10. Quince vacas _____ gestantes. _____ signos normales y _____ bien.

EXERCISE 4-2

Translate the following sentences from English to Spanish. Helpful hints:

- *Y* means "and."
- When "it" is the subject, just use the verb alone. For example: "It is pneumonia" translates as *Es neumonía*. "It is weak" translates as *Está débil*.
- Use the article instead of a possessive when talking about parts of the body. For example: "its tail" translates as *la cola*; "his ears" translates as *las orejas*.
- To make a sentence negative, put the word *no* in front of the verb. *El perro tiene sarna* (The dog has mange) becomes *El perro no tiene sarna* (The dog doesn't have mange).

- When you make a list of things to do, use the infinitive for each item rather than conjugating each verb separately. I'm going to take its temperature and listen to its heart: *Voy a tomar la temperatura y escuchar el corazón.*

1. The horse has colic. It's in pain, and it is seriously ill.
2. The cat has a fever, and its eyes are sunken.
3. I'm going to do some tests. Then (*Entonces*) I'm going to consult a specialist.
4. Spot is better! His temperature is normal.
5. The cow is pregnant, but (*pero*) it is weak and a little thin.
6. The dogs have distemper. They're very sick.
7. The lesion is better, but it is still a little inflamed.
8. The calf has difficulty breathing, and its mucus is green.
9. Mr. González is the owner of a modern dairy. He is an esteemed client. He is intelligent and nice, too. I'm going to examine his (*sus*) cows tomorrow.
10. Pooky is not seriously ill. He has parasites, but this pill will eliminate the parasites. In a week (*semana*), he will be fine.
11. I'm going to bandage the wound and prescribe some pills.
12. The specialist will go over the test results and recommend a treatment.

EXERCISE 4-3

Describe the symptoms of the following conditions in Spanish. Example: *La vaca tiene neumonía; tiene tos.* (The cow has pneumonia; it has a cough.) Include as many symptoms as you can.

1. El carnero tiene reticulopericarditis traumática.
2. El cerdo tiene neumonía.
3. La gata tiene falla renal.
4. El caballo tiene cólico.
5. La vaca tiene mastitis.

EXERCISE 4-4

Translate the following sentences from English to Spanish.

1. This medicine will cure the problem. (Note: For "will," use the Spanish version of "is going to.")
   This medicine should cure the problem.
   This medicine can cure the problem.

2. We can return tomorrow.
   We have to return tomorrow.
   We are going to return tomorrow.

3. I will take some x-rays.
   I need to take some x-rays.
   I have just taken some x-rays.
   I have to take some x-rays.

World's Simplest Verb: *hay*

And then there is the world's simplest irregular verb: *hay* (pronounced like the English word "eye"). It only has one form; it never changes. It means "there is" or "there are." Examples:

Hay una solución fácil. [**There is an easy solution.**]
No hay una solución fácil. [**There isn't an easy solution.**]
Hay tres moscas en la sopa. [**There are three flies in the soup.**]

EXERCISE 4-5

Translate the following sentences from English to Spanish.

1. There is a problem.
2. There are five cows with brucellosis.
3. There is blood in the urine.
4. There are no signs of leukemia.
5. There is a new medicine for this condition.

CHAPTER 5

How Long Has the Cow Had a Fever?

Duration of Time

One of the important questions that a veterinarian asks a client is how long the animal has had the symptoms. The first step in learning how to express this idea is to learn a few vocabulary words.

el minuto	**minute**
la hora	**hour**
el día	**day**
la semana	**week**
el mes	**month**
el año	**year**

The next step is to use the verb *hacer* (to make, to do). We'll get into the full use of *hacer* in another chapter. But for this chapter it is important to know that its impersonal form is *hace* (it makes). Put this together with a time phrase, a verb, and *que*, and you've got the length of time something has gone on or its duration.

Hace dos días que el perro tiene diarrea. [**The dog has had diarrhea for two days now. (Literally, it makes two days that the dog has diarrhea.)**]

Hace una semana que la cabra tiene hematuria. [**The goat has had hematuria for a week now. (It makes a week that the goat has hematuria.)**]

Notice that the concept of "now" is understood in this formula; you don't have to actually say it.

To elicit information about time duration, here is the question you'll ask your client:

¿Cuánto tiempo hace que el animal tiene estos signos? [**How long has the animal had these symptoms?**]

It's quite likely that the client won't answer with a complete sentence. Instead, a short phrase will do just fine. *"¿Cuánto tiempo hace que tiene estos signos?" "Dos días"* or *"Hace dos días."*

Here are some examples of information that your clients may tell you.

Hace una semana que la vaca tiene tos. [**The cow has been coughing for a week.**]

Hace doce horas que el caballo tiene respiración dificultosa. [**The horse has been wheezing for twelve hours.**]

Hace dos días que el loro está enfermo. [**The parrot has been sick for two days.**]

EXERCISE 5-1

Answer the question, expressing the idea of duration.

1. ¿Cuánto tiempo hace que el caballo sufre de cólico? (un día)
2. ¿Cuánto tiempo hace que la orina está sanguinolenta? (unos pocos días)
3. ¿Cuánto tiempo hace que la gata tiene la lesíon? (una semana)
4. ¿Cuánto tiempo hace que el toro no come? (tres días)
5. ¿Cuánto tiempo hace que la oveja trata de parir? (doce horas)
6. ¿Cuánto tiempo hace que el canario tiene parásitos? (dos semanas)
7. ¿Cuánto tiempo hace que tiene el tumor? (un mes, más o menos)

The Present Perfect

You may have noticed that the English equivalents of the duration sentences already used in this chapter are not in the present tense. This is one of the differences between English and Spanish. Duration in Spanish is expressed with the present tense, whereas duration in English is usually expressed with the present perfect. The perfect verbs are not pure or flawless; *per fect* in Latin means "already done." These verbs refer to things that have already occurred. The present perfect is the verb that talks about things that started before now, previous to the present moment. Here are some examples in English.

The cat <u>has shown</u> signs of leukemia.
Lately, the pig <u>has coughed</u> more.
I <u>have isolated</u> the cow.

To make the present perfect in Spanish, you need two parts, just as in English. First, there is the verb *haber* (to have, not the sense of *tener*, which is to own). Here are its forms (don't pronounce the *h*!).

yo he	*nosotros hemos*
tú has	
él, ella, usted ha	*ellos, ellas, ustedes han*

Put one of these forms together with the participle, which is formed by breaking off the *-ar*, *-er*, or *-ir* of the infinitive and adding *-ado* or *-ido*.

notar becomes *notado*
comer becomes *comido*
añadir becomes *añadido*

Now put it all together:

¿Ha notado usted un cambio? [**Have you noticed a change?**]
No ha comido hoy. [**It (the animal) has not eaten today.**]
No hemos añadido más calcio. [**We have not added more calcium.**]

EXERCISE 5-2

Translate these sentences into Spanish, using the present perfect of the verb in parentheses.

1. *(mejorar)* The parrot has improved a little.
2. *(vomitar)* The dog has not vomited today.
3. *(cojear)* The mare has limped since then *[desde entonces]*.
4. *(perder)* The kittens have lost weight.
5. *(crecer)* The cyst has grown.
6. *(desaparecer)* The mites have almost disappeared.
7. *(revisar)* I have checked over the results.
8. *(parir)* The sow has given birth.
9. *(disminuir)* The swelling has shrunk.
10. *(ayudar)* The vitamins have helped a lot.

EXERCISE 5-3

Translate the following paragraph into Spanish. You'll need to use the present perfect in some phrases, and in others, you'll use the present and the *hace que* duration expression.

Happy has been sick for almost six days. For three days, he hasn't eaten much, and he has vomited twice, but he has drunk a lot of water. Today he has not eaten, and it's been five hours that he has not urinated. I think that his condition has worsened.

The Verb *dar*

Another useful verb is *dar* (to give). Here it is conjugated in the present tense:

yo doy	*nosotros damos*
tú das	
él, ella, usted da	*ellos, ellas, ustedes dan*

This verb is often combined with *le* to indicate the person or thing that receives whatever is being given. For example, here's a question you'll be asking your clients:

¿Qué le da de comer? [**What do you give it to eat?**]

The client might answer with:

> *Le doy el heno.* [**I give it hay.**]
> *Le doy el alpiste.* [**I give it birdseed.**]

For more than one animal, change *le* to *les*.

> *¿Qué les da de comer?* [**What do you give them to eat?**]
> *Les doy el heno.* [**I give them hay.**]
> *Les doy el alpiste.* [**I give them birdseed.**]

The verb *dar* works well with infinitive phrases, too.

> *Voy a darle menos pipas.* [**I'm going to give it fewer sunflower seeds.**]
> *Usted debe darle menos pipas.* [**You should give it fewer sunflower seeds.**]
> *Usted necesita darle menos pipas.* [**You need to give it fewer sunflower seeds.**]

And, of course, *dar* can be put into the present perfect as well.

> *No les hemos dado suplementos.* [**We haven't given them supplements.**]
> *¿Le ha dado usted las verduras frescas?* [**Have you given it fresh vegetables?**]

Mi esposo le ha dado sobras de comida. [**My husband has given it table scraps.**]

Feeding Vocabulary

Here are some more things that you might feed an animal.

alfalfa	la alfalfa
apples	las manzanas
barley	la cebada
birdseed	el alpiste
bonemeal	la harina de huesos
brewer's yeast	la levadura de cerveza
canned food	la comida enlatada
carrots	las zanahorias
cereal	el cereal
clover	el trébol
cod liver oil	el aceite de hígado de bacalao
corn	el maíz
cottonseed cake	la torta de algodón
dry food	la comida desecada, la comida seca
grass	el pasto, la hierba
grit	el grit
hay	el heno
iodine	el yodo
milk	la leche
millet	el mijo, el millo
molasses	la melaza
oats	la avena
oilcake	la torta oleaginosa
ryegrass	el ballico, el ryegrass
salt	la sal
sedum	la hierba callera
seeds	las semillas
sorghum	el sorgo
supplements	los suplementos
table scraps	las sobras de comida
treats	los premios, las galletitas, las botanas, los obsequios
vegetables	las verduras

vetch	la veza
vitamins	las vitaminas
wet food	la comida húmeda

Other feeding-related terms:

amino acid	el aminoácido
balanced diet	la dieta balanceada
calcium	el calcio
daily feed	la alimentación diaria
feed trough	el comedero
forage	el forraje
grazing	el pastoreo
indigestion	la indigestión
iron deficiency	la carencia de hierro
magnesium deficiency	la carencia de magnesio
malnutrition	la desnutrición
overfeed	sobrealimentar
pastured animals	los animales a pasto
refusal to eat	la aversión por el alimento
silage	el ensilaje
stabled animals	los animales estabulados

EXERCISE 5-4

Translate the following sentences into Spanish. Notice that some are in the present, some use infinitive phrases, and some are in the present perfect.

1. We have not given vitamins to the kittens.
2. You should not overfeed your animal.
3. It is suffering from iron deficiency.
4. I want to give it a balanced diet.
5. Can we give it treats?
6. Mister García, do you give it dry food or canned food?
7. What supplements have you given it?
8. I have fed them corn until *(hasta)* this year.
9. What should we feed it?
10. It has had indigestion for two days now.

EXERCISE 5-5

Answer the following questions with a complete sentence.

1. ¿Cuánto tiempo hace que la vaca tiene aversión por el alimento?
2. ¿Les da vitaminas a los cerdos?

3. Señor Vargas, ¿qué le da de comer a su ganado?
4. Los caballos, ¿están a pasto o estabulados?
5. ¿Qué ha comido el macho cabrió que le causa tanta indigestión?
6. Señor Sánchez, ¿en qué consiste la comida diaria de su perro?
7. ¿Cuántos *(How many)* obsequios le da usted?
8. Señora Navarro, ¿les da a las vacas suficiente sal?

Listening for Key Phrases

Often, when you ask a client a question, you'll get a long complicated answer. For example, if you ask how long the dog has had this swelling, the answer could be something like this: "Well, I'm not sure exactly. The first time I became aware of it was when my in-laws were visiting from Florida. They noticed it when they were playing with the dog. I guess that was about two weeks ago, more or less." When you get an answer like that in your own language, you probably only hear "not sure exactly . . . two weeks ago." We don't really listen carefully to each other, and we certainly don't hear every word! Instead, we use a filtering system that I call "the pearl in the mud." Our hearing ignores the mud and focuses on the pearl, that is, the answer to the question. In the previous example, the pearl is "two weeks ago." All the rest is mud. Your response to the statement would not be, "Oh, your in-laws live in Florida?" It would be, "Has it grown in the last two weeks?"

In Spanish, you should use the same filtering system. Don't panic when the client gives you a long response that you don't understand. Look for the phrase or word that tells you the answer you want. Often, a long response begins with *sí* or *no*, which may be the only word you really need. If you were given the preceding response, all you would need to listen for is *hace dos semanas*. Don't worry about the in-laws in Florida.

Many English speakers think that Spanish is spoken rapidly. In most cases, that's only because they don't understand it; the actual speed is no different from that of English. Keep in mind that Spanish speakers think that English is spoken rapidly, too. If you want to help out a Spanish-speaking friend who is learning English, put spaces between your words. Don't say, "Howareyoutoday?"; say, "How are you today?" The friend may be sufficiently grateful to speak that way in Spanish with you. This seems like a good place to introduce the phrase *Hable más despacio, por favor.* (Speak more slowly, please.)

CHAPTER 6

The Past and Accidents

Past Time Verbs

Your clients will often tell you about their animals' accidents and sudden illnesses. These things usually occurred in the past: "Last night the cow suddenly started to cough and wheeze," or "Yesterday the fever rose." Linguists call the verb form or tense that conveys this idea the preterite, but we'll call it, surprisingly enough, the past. Here are its endings:

revisar [**to review, to check, to check over**]

revisé [**I checked**]	*revisamos* [**we checked**]
revisaste [**you (informal) checked**]	
revisó [**she, he, you (formal) checked**]	*revisaron* [**they, you all checked**]

toser [**to cough**]

tosí [**I coughed**]	*tosimos* [**we coughed**]
tosiste [**you (informal) coughed**]	
tosió [**she, he, you (formal) coughed**]	*tosieron* [**they, you all coughed**]

vivir [**to live**]

viví [**I lived**]	*vivimos* [**we lived**]
viviste [**you (informal) lived**]	
vivió [**she, he, you (formal) lived**]	*vivieron* [**they, you all lived**]

Words or Phrases That Indicate Time

Present and future time
hoy (**today**)
esta noche (**tonight**)
mañana (**tomorrow**)
la próxima semana (**next week**)
este año (**this year**)
ahora (**now**)

Past time
ayer (**yesterday**)
anoche (**last night**)
esta mañana (**this morning**)
la semana pasada (**last week**)
el año pasado (**last year**)
entonces (**then**)

EXERCISE 6-1

Fill in the blank with the appropriate form of the past tense.

1. Hace dos días que la vaca _____ (parir) con dificultad.
2. Los chivos _____ (recibir) las vacunas en febrero.
3. Anoche mi hijo [my son] _____ (descubrir) la fractura.
4. Manuel _____ (observar) el problema cuando _____ (ordeñar) las vacas esta mañana.
5. El doctor Méndez _____ (diagnosticar) la brucelosis y los dueños de la granja _____ (eliminar) los animales infectados. _____ (vacunar) los demás [the rest].
6. El destete [weaning] de los corderos se _____ (realizar) a los noventa [ninety] días de edad.
7. Yo _____ (desinfectar) y _____ (vendar) la herida.
8. La semana pasada, María y yo _____ (evaluar) el rebaño y _____ (decidir) comprar ocho cabras.
9. El toro no _____ (presentar) defecto físico, pero ultimamente no _____ (mostrar) interés sexual para la monta.
10. Hace una semana que usted _____ (bañar) los animales contra los parásitos externos, ¿verdad?
11. Ayer la veterinaria _____ (someter) los cachorros a las pruebas de sangre.
12. La semana pasada el loro _____ (parecer) nervioso y se _____ (picar) su plumaje.
13. ¿_____ (revisar) usted los rayos x del gato de la señora Espinoza?
14. Hace dos meses que nosotros _____ (añadir) el hierro a su dieta.
15. Anoche la fiebre _____ (subir) mucho.

What About the Weak-Kneed Verbs?

Most weak-kneed verbs do not show change in the past because the stress is on the ending.

perder (ie) [**to lose**]

perdí	*perdimos*
perdiste	
perdió	*perdieron*

Some weak-kneed verbs are still weak, even in the past tense, but only in the third person. These verbs are noted with two changes in parentheses: the first for the present tense, the second for the past tense.

sugerir (i, i) [**to suggest**]

sugerí	*sugerimos*
sugeriste	
sugirió	*sugirieron*

EXERCISE 6-2

Write the present and the past of the following weak-kneed verbs, according to the indicated subject.

Example: *los rayos x + probar* (ue) should be *prueban, probaron.*

1. el gato + empezar (ie)
2. los especialistas + recomendar (ie)
3. el potrillo + dormir (ue, u)
4. el perro + morder (ue)
5. la paloma + volar (ue)
6. las llamas + seguir (i, i)
7. el maíz + costar (ue)
8. el laboratorio + pedir (i, i)
9. los canarios + morir (ue, u)
10. el problema + volver (ue)

What, No Irregular Verbs?

Alas, there are quite a few irregular past-tense verbs. Listed here are some of the most useful ones.

ser [**to be**] and *ir* [**to go**]

fui	*fuimos*
fuiste	
fue	*fueron*

(Yes, they have the same conjugation in the past. No, we don't know why.)

hacer [**to do, to make**]

hice	*hicimos*
hiciste	
hizo	*hicieron*

estar [**to be,** used with changeable conditions]

estuve	*estuvimos*
estuviste	
estuvo	*estuvieron*

tener [**to have, to own**]

tuve	*tuvimos*
tuviste	
tuvo	*tuvieron*

dar [**to give**]

di	*dimos*
diste	
dio	*dieron*

Here's what these verbs look like in a sentence:

Fue un parto difícil. [**It was a difficult birth.**]

No hice mucho porque el cordero murió antes de mi llegada. [**I didn't do much because the lamb died before my arrival.**]

Le di hierro y vitaminas. [**I gave it iron and vitamins.**]

La gata estuvo mejor hasta esta mañana. [**The cat was better until this morning.**]

EXERCISE 6-3

Translate the following sentences into Spanish, using the present and past tenses of the verb.

1. (*dar*) I give it molasses. I gave it molasses.
2. (*ser*) The discharge is abundant. The discharge was abundant.
3. (*estar*) The situation is grave. The situation became grave.
4. (*hacer*) Exercise makes the problem worse. Exercise made the problem worse.
5. (*tener*) They have regular vaccinations. They had (received) regular vaccinations.

Now that you know the past tense, you can talk about events in the present, the present perfect, the past, and the future. Here's an example:

Gana peso normalmente. [**It (the animal) gains weight normally.**]
Ha ganado peso normalmente. [**It has gained weight normally.**]
Ganó peso normalmente. [**It gained weight normally.**]
Va a ganar peso normalmente. [**It will gain weight normally.**]

EXERCISE 6-4

Translate the following sentences into Spanish, noticing the time frame of each one.

1. (*examinar*) I examine Mr. Vivaldi's flock every year.
   I'm going to examine Mr. Vivaldi's flock tomorrow.
   I examined Mr. Vivaldi's flock yesterday.
   I have already examined Mr. Vivaldi's flock.

2. (*mostrar, ue*) The tests have shown lack of magnesium.
   The tests show lack of magnesium.
   The tests showed lack of magnesium.
   The tests will show lack of magnesium.

3. (*expulsar*) This medicine gets rid of the parasites.
   This medicine got rid of the parasites.
   This medicine will get rid of the parasites.
   This medicine has gotten rid of the parasites.

4. (*dar*) Now we give it an injection.
   Last week, we gave it an injection.
   After this [después], we will give it an injection.
   We have given it an injection.

5. (*comer*) It eats normally now.
   It ate normally until yesterday.
   Today, it has eaten normally.
   It will eat normally soon.

Accidents

There is a special way of discussing accidents that happen out of the blue. In these cases, you aren't focusing on the culprit or the initiator of the action. You focus instead on saying that it happened to the animal. In this formula, the phrase consists of three parts: *se*, *le*, and a verb in the past.

Example: *Se le fracturó la pierna.* (Literally, the leg broke itself for him. In English it means, he broke his leg, or it broke its leg.)

¿Qué le pasó? or *¿Qué le sucedió?* [**What happened (to the animal)?**]
   Se le rompió la pierna. [**It broke its leg.**]
   Se le infectó la pezuña. [**Its hoof got infected.**]
   Se le infectaron los ojos. [**Its eyes got infected.**]

Other verbs just use the *se* and the past verb form. Notice that the focus in these examples is on something the animal did, rather than on something that happened to the animal.

Se tragó un clavo. [**She swallowed a nail.**]
   Se cayó en el arroyo. [**It fell in a ditch.**]
   Se cortó con un alambre. [**He cut himself on barbed wire.**]
   Se mordió un cable eléctrico. [**It bit/chewed an electrical wire.**]
   Se peleó con el gato de mi vecino. [**She had a fight with my neighbor's cat.**]
   Se tomó veneno. [**He drank poison.**]

But when you want to identify the perpetrator, don't use *se*. In the following examples, the focus is on someone who took action on the animal.

Le dispararon unos muchachos. [**Some kids shot him.**]
   Le mordió ese gato que tiene mi vecino. [**That cat of my neighbor bit her.**]
   Le atropelló un auto. [**He got hit by a car.**]
   Mi nietita le dio chocolates. [**My little granddaughter gave it chocolates.**]

EXERCISE 6-5

Translate these sentences into Spanish.

1. It swallowed a wire.
2. The wound got infected.
3. It fell in a hole (hole in the ground—*el hoyo*).
4. It cut itself on a nail.
5. It broke its rib.
6. It drank antifreeze.
7. It was run over by a motorcycle (*la motocicleta*).
8. It was bitten by a snake. [Note: With snakes, use *picar* instead of *morder.*]
9. It damaged its wing.
10. My little grandson gave it aspirin (*la aspirina*).

CHAPTER 7

Telling People What to Do

Verbal Shorthand

We don't always repeat the name of something every time we say it. For example, what is wrong with this conversation?

"Dad, do you have the newspaper?"

"No, I don't have the newspaper. Perhaps your mother has the newspaper."

"I already asked her about the newspaper. She says you have the newspaper."

Too many "newspapers!" We don't talk like this. Instead, once we've identified the object, we use a shorthand form for it. Here is a more realistic dialogue:

"Dad, do you have the newspaper?"

"No, I don't have it. Perhaps your mother has it."

"I already asked her about it. She says you have it."

In this case, "it" is the shorthand way of saying "newspaper." Once the word "newspaper" is used, "it" can take its place subsequently, as long as you are still speaking to the same person. But if you leave Dad to go talk to Mom, you'll have to mention "newspaper" once, so that she'll know what you're talking about.

Here are some handy shorthand forms in Spanish:

me	me ("me" and *me* are not pronounced the same way!)
te	you (informal)
lo	you (formal, for a man), it (for a masculine noun)
la	you (formal, for a woman), it (for a feminine noun)

nos	us
los	you all, you guys, you (plural, masculine), them (masculine)
las	you all, you gals, you (plural, feminine), them (feminine)

In a sentence, the shorthand form, or pronoun, goes right before the verb.

Lo tengo. [**I have it; referring to *el ungüento* (the ointment)**]

Elena la vendió. [**Elena bandaged it; referring to *la llaga* (the sore or the ulcer)**]

Las comió. [**He ate them; referring to *las semillas* (the seeds)**]

If the sentence has a negative sense, the *no* goes in front of the shorthand.

No lo tengo. [**I don't have it.**]

Elena no la vendió. [**Elena didn't bandage it.**]

No las comió. [**He didn't eat them.**]

EXERCISE 7-1

Answer the question with a positive and a negative.

Example: *¿Tiene usted el termómetro?* [**Do you have the thermometer?**]

Sí, lo tengo. [**Yes, I have it.**]

No, no lo tengo. [**No, I don't have it.**]

1. ¿Tiene fiebre? (a question while examining a cow)
2. ¿Toman vitaminas? (examining piglets)
3. ¿Come alpiste? (examining a canary)
4. ¿Receta usted antibióticos en estos casos?
5. ¿Desinfectó usted el ombligo?
6. ¿Pesó usted las ovejas?
7. Y el gato, ¿toma alguna medicina?
8. ¿Tiene dificultad cuando orina? (examining the dog)
9. ¿Ha notado usted algun cambio?
10. Las cabras, ¿recibieron las vacunas normales?

Giving Commands

A normal part of conversation consists of giving polite commands, such as "Pick me up at eight," "Tell me what he said," and "Pass the salt, please." Veterinarians also use commands such as "Hold the cow while I inject this," "Give it three pills a day," or "Take the animal's temperature, and call me if it goes up again."

These requests are formed by using switched endings. You have previously learned that -*ar* verbs use endings that incorporate the letter *a*, and that -*er* and -*ir* endings incorporate the letter *e*. Well, for commands, it's the opposite, and you use *e* for -*ar* verbs and *a* for -*er* and -*ir* verbs.

Here are some examples (the command form of the verb is underlined):

hablar [**to speak**]
Hable más despacio, por favor. [**Speak more slowly, please.**]

leer [**to read**]
Lea las instrucciones con cuidado. [**Read the directions carefully.**]

añadir [**to add**]
Añada este suplemento a su dieta. [**Add this supplement to its diet.**]

Weak-Kneed Commands

The weak-kneed verbs will show their change in the command form (the command form of the verb is underlined).

volver (ue) [**to come back**]
Vuelva usted mañana. [**Come back tomorrow.**]

extender (ie) [**to extend**]
Extienda el ala, por favor. [**Extend its wing, please.**]

Negative Commands

If you want to make a negative command, just put *no* in front of the verb.

No olvide. [**Don't forget.**]
No espere. [**Don't wait.**]
No mueva la pierna. [**Don't move its leg.**]

EXERCISE 7-2

Fill in the blank with the proper form of the command verb.

1. _____ (esperar) un momento, por favor.
2. _____ (doblar) la pierna del caballo.
3. Doctora Fernández, _____ (tomar) la temperatura, por favor.
4. No _____ (añadir) más sal a su dieta.
5. Julio, _____ (describir) los síntomas, por favor.
6. _____ (abrir) la botella, por favor.
7. _____ (proceder) de la siguiente manera.
8. _____ (leer) con cuidado las precauciones en la etiqueta.
9. No _____ (olvidar) las vitaminas.

10. No _____ (cambiar) la venda.

11. _____ (empezar [ie]) el tratamiento mañana.

12. No _____ (volver [ue]) usted si no hay problemas.

Irregular Commands

Just to keep things lively, there are some common irregular commands. These you'll just have to memorize.

> *tener* [**to have**]
> *Tenga cuidado con los pesticidas.* [**Be careful with pesticides.**]
>
> *hacer* [**to do, to make**]
> *Haga lo posible.* [**Do what you can.**]
>
> *decir* [**to tell, to say**]
> *Diga las direcciones lentamente.* [**Tell/Say the directions slowly.**]
>
> *poner* [**to put**]
> *Ponga el heno en el suelo.* [**Put the hay on the floor.**]
>
> *ser* [**to be**]
> *Sea profesional con sus clientes.* [**Be professional with your clients.**]
>
> *estar* [**to be**]
> *Esté tranquilo, la cerda va a sobrevivir.* [**Be calm, the sow will live.**]
>
> *ir* [**to go**]
> *Vaya a la farmacia Cruz Roja.* [**Go to the Red Cross pharmacy.**]
>
> *seguir* [**to follow**]
> *Siga con el tratamiento.* [**Stay with/Keep doing the treatment.**]
>
> *dar* [**to give**]
> *Dé menos premios.* [**Give fewer treats.**]

The command verbs act like magnets when they're positive. They attract words like *me* and *lo*. In that case, the word sticks to the end of the command. But they repel those words when they're negative, so that the word is not part of the command. Note the following positive and negative forms of *hacer*.

> Positive: *Hágalo.* [**Do it.**]
> Negative: *No lo haga.* [**Don't do it.**]

EXERCISE 7-3

Express the following ideas in Spanish, using both a positive and a negative form.

> *olvidar* [**to forget**]
> Forget it. Don't forget it.
> *Olvídelo. No lo olvide.*

1. (*decir*) Tell me. Don't tell me.
2. (*poner*) Put them (*los rayos x*) here (*aquí*). Don't put them here.
3. (*tomar*) Take it (*la temperatura*). Don't take it.
4. (*inyectar*) Inject it (*la vacuna*). Don't inject it.
5. (*describir*) Describe them (*los signos*). Don't describe them.

Giving Something to Somebody

Imagine that you are giving a gift to Manuel. You are the subject, the person doing the action. The gift is the object, the thing that is being passed from one person to the other. Manuel is the lucky receiver of the gift. To indicate that someone or something is the receiver (also called the indirect object), use one of these receiving words:

me me (Note the difference in pronunciation!)
te you (informal)
le you (formal), him, her, or it
nos us
les you (plural), them

EXERCISE 7-4

In the following sentences, underline the receiver.

1. Give the goat a carrot.
2. Give it more salt.
3. Tell me the problem.
4. Write him a report.
5. Inject it with the vaccine.

The receiving words function like the shorthand words you've already learned. Here are some examples.

Dele una zanahoria a la cabra. [**Give the goat a carrot.**]
No le dé una zanahoria a la cabra. [**Don't give the goat a carrot.**]
Dele más sal. [**Give it more salt.**]
No le dé más sal. [**Don't give it more salt.**]
Dígame el problema. [**Tell me the problem.**]
No me diga el problema. [**Don't tell me the problem.**]
Escríbale un informe. [**Write him a report.**]
No le escriba un informe. [**Don't write him a report.**]
Inyéctele la vacuna. [**Inject it with the vaccine.**]
No le inyecte la vacuna. [**Don't inject it with the vaccine.**]

Express the following ideas involving receivers in Spanish.

1. (*dar*) Give it a pill every day.
2. (*decir*) Tell him the problem.
3. (*describir*) Describe the symptoms to me.
4. (*pasar*) Pass me the thermometer, please.
5. (*mostrar, ue*) Show me the sore.
6. (*dar*) Don't give them table scraps.
7. (*recetar*) Don't prescribe antibiotics for it yet.

Polite Suggestions

As useful as commands are, you don't want to use them excessively or run the risk of appearing brusque or rude. So here's another way to give a command, but this time in the form of a suggestion. You still use the command form, but you express it in an indirect way. In the indirect form, the receiving words and the shorthand words don't stick to the verb, they go in front of it:

Direct command: *Dele más vitaminas.* [**Give it more vitamins.**]

Indirect command: *Sugiero que usted le dé más vitaminas.* [**I suggest that you give it more vitamins.**]

Both the direct and the indirect commands are proper grammatically, and they are both polite culturally. But the suggestion is a little less emphatic than the command. Learn to use both ways. Here are some suggestion phrases.

Sugiero que . . . [**I suggest that . . .**]
No sugiero que . . . [**I don't suggest that . . .**]
Recomiendo que . . . [**I recommend that . . .**]
No recomiendo que . . . [**I don't recommend that . . .**]
Es necesario que . . . [**It is necessary that . . .**]
No es necesario que . . . [**It is not necessary that . . .**]
Prefiero que . . . [**I prefer that . . .**]
Es importante que . . . [**It is important that . . .**]

Translate the following sentences into Spanish.

1. (*limpiar*) It is important that you clean them [*los dientes*] regularly.
2. (*pasar la noche*) It is not necessary that Patches spend the night in the clinic.

3. (*consultar*) I recommend that you consult with a veterinary opthamologist.
4. (*tomar*) The specialist suggests that we take x-rays.
5. (*desinfectar*) It is important that you disinfect the navel.
6. (*cambiar*) I don't recommend that you change its diet.
7. (*rasgar*) It is important that it doesn't scratch the wound.
8. (*cubrir*) I suggest that you cover the area with ointment.
9. (*lamer*) It is important that Maddie doesn't lick it [*la llaga*].
10. (*perder, ie*) It is necessary that Bubbles lose weight.

Some Common Commands

Give it one of these pills three times a day for ten days.	Dele una de estas pastillas tres veces al día por diez días.
Keep it away from other animals.	Manténgalo separado de otros animales.
Take stool samples.	Tome muestras de excremento.
Watch it closely.	Obsérvelo con atención.
Keep it in a corral.	Manténgalo en un corral.
Keep it in a dry stall.	Manténgalo en una caseta seca.
Don't put it in the pasture.	No lo saque a la pastura.
Don't let it graze.	No lo deje pastar.
Clean the wound.	Limpie la herida.
Apply this ointment.	Aplique este ungüento.
Apply this powder.	Aplique este polvo.
Change the bandages.	Cambie los vendajes.
Give it an injection once a day for five days.	Dele una inyección una vez al día por cinco días.
If the symptoms return, give me a call.	Si los signos vuelven, llámeme.
Come back in a week.	Regrese/Vuelva en una semana.
Bathe the animal in this solution.	Bañe al animal en esta disolución.

Squirt this in its mouth.	Introduzca esto por la boca.
Put these drops in its eye.	Ponga estas gotas en el ojo.
Give it this special food.	Dele este alimento especial.
Add calcium to its diet.	Adicione/Añada calcio a su dieta.

CHAPTER 8

Taking a Clinical History

One of the first things you'll do when meeting a client is to take a clinical history of the client's animal. The following questions will help you in this first step. Make a flash card for each one. Ask yourself, "What would be a logical answer for this question?"

The preliminary facts [*Los datos preliminares*]

Is it male or female?	¿Es macho o hembra?
How old is it?	¿Qué edad tiene?
What breed is it?	¿Qué raza es?
What do you feed it?	¿Qué le da de comer?
How many births has it had?	¿Cuántos partos ha tenido?
How much does it weigh?	¿Cuánto pesa?
What vaccinations has it had?	¿Qué vacunas se le han puesto?
Is it pastured or stabled?	¿Está a pasto o estabulado?
Did you acquire it recently?	¿Lo consiguió recientemente?
Where?	¿Dónde?
How many animals do you have in total?	¿Cuántos animales tiene en total?
What other animals are on the farm or in the house?	¿Qué otras especies hay en la granja o en la casa?
Have there been new animals introduced to the farm or house?	¿Ha introducido nuevos animales a la granja o la casa?

Preliminary description of the problem
[Descripción preliminar del problema]

What's wrong with your animal?	¿Qué le pasa a su animal?
When did the problem start?	¿Cuándo comenzó el problema?
How long has it had this problem?	¿Cuánto tiempo hace que tiene este problema?
Has it had this problem before?	¿Ha tenido este problema anteriormente?
Is it taking any medication?	¿Toma algún medicamento?
Has it lost weight?	¿Ha perdido peso?
Does it have an appetite?	¿Tiene apetito?
Have the symptoms worsened?	¿Han empeorado los signos?
How many animals are affected?	¿Cuántos animales están afectados?
Have you noticed any change in the animal's habits or behavior?	¿Ha notado algún cambio en los hábitos del animal o en el comportamiento?
Did it begin suddenly or gradually?	¿Comenzó repentinamente o gradualmente?
Is it pregnant?	¿Está preñada?
Have they eaten anything unusual or new?	¿Han comido algo extraño o nuevo?
Have they been out of the region, state, or country?	¿Han estado fuera de la región, el estado, o el país?

Talking with the client [Conversando con el cliente/la cliente]

I'd like to ask you some questions.	Quisiera hacerle unas preguntas.
I'm going to . . .	Voy a . . .
take its temperature.	tomar su temperatura.
do a blood test.	hacer un examen sanguíneo.
listen to its breathing.	escuchar su respiración.
listen to its heart.	escuchar su ritmo cardíaco.
take an x-ray.	tomar unos rayos x.
take a biopsy.	sacar una biopsia.

Let's see.	Vamos a ver.
Don't worry.	No se preocupe.
I'm not sure.	No estoy segura/seguro.
The animal will be fine in a few days.	El animal estará bien en unos días.
I'm sorry, there's nothing that can be done.	Lo siento, no hay nada que se pueda hacer.
As a precaution, you should isolate the animal from the others.	Como precaución, debería aislar el animal de los otros.
There's a simple solution to this problem.	Hay una solución sencilla para este problema.
Please wait in the waiting room.	Por favor, espere en la sala de espera.
I'll be with you shortly.	Estaré con usted pronto.
Please hold your animal still (small animals).	Sostenga a su animal, por favor.
Restrain your animal please (large animals).	Sujete a su animal, por favor.

The Diagnostic Exam

Here are some questions to ask when examining the animal. Note that they are designed to elicit easy-to-understand answers, such as "yes" and "no." Simple, no?

The cardiopulmonary system [*El sistema cardiopulmonar*]

Does it cough?	¿Tiene tos?
Does it cough up any phlegm?	¿Tose con flema?

What color is the phlegm?
  clear
  white
  yellow
  green
  dark
  brown
  tinged with blood
	¿De qué color es la flema?
	  clara
	  blanca
	  amarilla
	  verde
	  oscura
	  marrón
	  manchada de sangre

Does it have trouble breathing?	¿Tiene dificultad para respirar?
Have you noticed any unusual sound in its breathing?	¿Ha notado algún sonido raro al respirar?
Does it tire easily?	¿Se cansa facilmente?
Does it have irregular breathing?	¿Tiene respiración irregular? ¿Tiene respiración agitada?
Does it have a nasal discharge?	¿Tiene escurrimiento nasal?
Does it breathe through the mouth?	¿Respira por la boca?

The cardiopulmonary system *(continued)*

Does it appear painful to breathe?	¿Muestra dolor al respirar?

The gastrointestinal system [*El sistema gastrointestinal*]

Does it have diarrhea? Is it frequent? Sporadic?	¿Tiene diarrea? ¿Es frecuente? ¿Esporádica?
Have you noticed any blood or mucus in the feces?	¿Ha notado sangre o mucosidad en las heces?
Does it vomit?	¿Tiene vómito?
Does food fall from its mouth?	¿Cae el alimento de la boca?
Does it have a problem chewing?	¿Tiene dificultad para masticar?
Does it lick things?	¿Lame objetos?
Is the abdomen distended?	¿Está distendido el abdomen?
Are the feces dry? Hard?	¿Están las heces secas? ¿Duras?
Do the feces have undigested material?	¿Tienen las heces material no digerido?
Is there a bad odor in the feces?	¿Tienen las heces olor fétido?
Have you noticed any parasites in the feces?	¿Ha notado parásitos en las heces?

The urinary system [*El sistema urinario*]

Does your animal have trouble urinating?	¿Tiene su animal dificultad al orinar?
What color is the urine? yellow cloudy reddish	¿De qué color es la orina? amarilla turbia rojiza
Is there blood in the urine?	¿Hay sangre en la orina?
Does it urinate too often?	¿Orina con demasiada frecuencia?

Have you noticed pus in the urine?	¿Ha notado pus en la orina?
Does it have difficulty starting to urinate?	¿Tiene dificultad al comenzar a orinar?
Does it have difficulty maintaining a stream?	¿Tiene dificultad para mantener el chorro?
Does the urine have an odor?	¿Tiene olor la orina?
Have you noticed incontinence?	¿Presenta incontinencia?
Does he/she seem to have pain when urinating?	¿Presenta dolor al orinar?

The mouth, throat, ears, eyes, and skin
[*La boca, la garganta, los oídos, los ojos, la piel*]

Have you noticed any bleeding from the gums or mouth?	¿Ha notado si las encías o la boca le sangran?
Does it have swelling or lumps in the mouth?	¿Tiene alguna hinchazón o bola en la boca?
Does it have difficulty swallowing?	¿Tiene dificultad al tragar?
Has it had bleeding from the nose?	¿Ha sangrado por la nariz?
Have you noticed any secretion from the ears?	¿Ha notado alguna secreción por los oídos?
Have you noticed any redness or swelling in the eyes?	¿Ha notado los ojos enrojecidos o hinchados?
Does it have runny eyes?	¿Tiene secreción ocular?
Does it have sores or blisters?	¿Tiene llagas o ampollas?
Have you noticed any skin wounds?	¿Tiene alguna herida en la piel?
Have you noticed it scratching a lot?	¿Se rasca con frecuencia?

The mouth, throat, ears, eyes, and skin *(continued)*

Have you noticed any fleas/lice/ticks?	¿Ha notado pulgas/piojos/garrapatas?

The musculoskeletal system [*El sistema musculoesquelético*]

Does it have trouble getting up?	¿Tiene dificultad para levantarse?
Is it unable to get up?	¿Está tumbado sin poder levantarse?
Does it limp?	¿Cojea?
Does it favor one foot?	¿Se apoya más en una pata?
Is it in pain?	¿Le duele?
Are any of the feet inflamed/broken?	¿Tiene alguna pata inflamada/rota?
Does it walk weakly?	¿Camina con debilidad?
Is it active?	¿Hace ejercicio frecuentemente?
Does it have a hunched posture?	¿Camina encojido?
Are there any hard swellings in the muscles?	¿Tiene los músculos duros?

The nervous system [*El sistema nervioso*]

Does it have difficulty in walking?	¿Tiene dificultad al caminar?
Does it stagger?	¿Tiene vértigo?
Does it tremble?	¿Tiene temblores?
Has it had convulsions?	¿Ha tenido convulsiones?
Does it shake its head?	¿Sacude la cabeza?
Is it aggressive?	¿Está agresivo?
Have you noticed any rigidity?	¿Ha notado alguna rigidez?
Does it go around in circles?	¿Marcha en círculos?
Does it salivate excessively?	¿Tiene salivación excesiva?

Have you noticed any lack of coordination?	¿Presenta incoordinación?

The reproductive system [*El sistema reproductivo*]

Does it have a discharge (with pus) from the vagina?	¿Le supura la vagina?
Does it have a discharge (without pus) from the vagina?	¿Tiene secreciones vaginales?
Has it been in season?	¿Ha estado en celo?
Has it been pregnant?	¿Ha estado preñada?
How many times has it given birth?	¿Cuántos partos ha tenido?
Has it had any abortions?	¿Ha tenido abortos?
Does it have difficulty in giving birth?	¿Tiene dificultad para parir?
Has it given birth recently?	¿Ha parido recientemente?
Have you noticed any change in milk production?	¿Ha notado algún cambio en la producción de leche?
Has it had any stillbirths?	¿Ha tenido mortinatos?
Is there any secretion from the penis?	¿Hay secreción del pene?
Is there any swelling in the scrotum?	¿Hay inflamación del escroto?
At what stage of gestation did the abortion occur?	¿En qué etapa de la gestación ocurrió el aborto?

CHAPTER 10

Cattle

How am I going to learn all this vocabulary?
Calm down, it'll be all right. Here are some shortcuts to learning this material.

• First of all, you probably don't need to learn every single one of these terms. Certain diseases are more common than others. It is my sincerest hope that you won't see a case of anthrax, but you most certainly will see cases of mastitis and lameness, so learn that vocabulary first. Different regions will have their own peculiar problems. For example, if you practice in Hawaii, you probably won't see cases of frostbite, but you will see parasite problems. Keep handy a list of the common conditions you regularly see in your practice.

• If the English version of the disease's name is Latin, then the Spanish version will be Latin too. Just add *la* in front, change *y* to *i*, change *th* to *t*, change *ph* to *f*, pronounce the vowels in the Spanish way, and voila! You've got the Spanishized Latin. Here are some examples:

enterotoxemia: *la enterotoxemia*
dyphtheria: *la difteria*

• Learn the basic word, then add the appropriate adjective (which often looks like English anyway). For example, if you learn the word for "failure," *la falla,* then you can use it as the basis for lots of conditions:

la falla renal
la falla cardíaca
la falla respiratoria

Here's another example: learn the word for "prolapse," *el prolapso,* and then merrily add the collapsing parts:

el prolapso uterino
el prolapso vaginal
el prolapso rectal

• When you're talking with a client, you probably won't use the technical term anyway. Choose a simple way to describe the animal's problem; for example, all sorts of *-itis* conditions can be described as *una infección de . . .* (now put the infected part here).

una infección de la membrana sobre el ojo [conjunctivitis]
una infección del ubre [mastitis]
una infección de la piel [dermatitis]

Or you can say that the problem is an *enfermedad* [illness]:

La vaca tiene una enfermedad bacterial.
una enfermedad viral.
una enfermedad pulmonar.

In desperate moments, you can even say *problema:*

La vaca tiene un problema respiratorio.
un problema del hígado.
un problema de nutrición.

• As with verbs, the best way to learn the vocabulary you need is by making flash cards and practicing regularly with them.

Here's a comforting thought: vocabulary included here will not be repeated in the following chapters. For example, if you learn "liver disease" (*la enfermedad hepática*) now, you won't have to do it again later. Whew! Now that you've calmed down, here are some special vocabulary, diseases, and conditions for cattle.

Special Vocabulary ⸺⸺⸺⸺⸺⸺⸺⸺⸺⸺

Special vocabulary for cattle [*Vocabulario especial del ganado*]

bull	el toro
cow	la vaca
calf	el ternero, la ternera
heifer	la vaquilla
steer	el novillo
ox	el buey
cattle	el ganado
beef cattle	el ganado de carne
dairy cattle	el ganado de leche
feedlot cattle	el ganado estabulado

grazing cattle	el ganado en pastoreo
corral	el corral
parlor	la sala de ordeña
colostrum	el calostro
palpation	la palpación
water trough	el bebedero
to moo	mugir
to ruminate	rumiar
to charge	embestir
calf hutch	la becerrera
forage	el forraje
concentrate	el concentrado
[such as a medicine]	
silage	el ensilaje
molasses	la melaza
minerals	los minerales
dishorn	descornar (*ue*)
dipping bath	el baño de inmersión
branding	el marcaje
artificial insemination	la inseminación artificial

Illnesses

The blood, lymphatic, and cardiovascular system
[*El sistema sanguíneo, linfático y cardiovascular*]

anaplasmosis	la anaplasmosis
anemia	la anemia
arrhythmia	la arritmia
babesiosis	la babesiosis
bovine leukosis	la leucosis bovina
cardiac hypertrophy	la hipertrofia cardíaca
cardiac insufficiency and failure	la insuficiencia cardíaca y el fallo cardíaco
endocarditis	la endocarditis
eperythrozoonosis	la eperitrozoonosis
heart sounds and murmurs	los sonidos y murmullos cardíacos
hemolytic disease in newborn calves	la enfermedad hemolítica de los terneros

hydropericardium	el hidropericardio
myocarditis	la miocarditis

The digestive system [*El sistema digestivo*]

abdominal hernia	la hernia abdominal
abomasal ulcer	la úlcera abomasal
atresia	la atresia
bloat	el timpanismo
bovine liver abscess	el abceso hepático bovino
bovine viral diarrhea	la diarrea viral bovina
bovine winter dysentery	la disentería invernal bovina
campylobacteriosis	la campilobacteriosis
coccidiosis	la coccidiosis
constipation	la constipación
cryptosporidiosis	la criptosporidiosis
dietary abomasal impaction	la impactación abomasal
dilation and torsion of the abomasum	la dilatación y la torsión del abomaso
displacement of the abomasum	el desplazamiento del abomaso
enteric disease	la enfermedad entérica
enteritis	la enteritis
fluke infection	la fasciolasis
gastrointestinal parasites	los parásitos gastrointestinales
gastrointestinal ulcer	la úlcera gastrointestinal
grain overload	la impactación ruminal
liver disease	la enfermedad hepática
peritonitis	la peritonitis
ptylism	el ptialismo
rectal prolapse	el prolapso rectal
salmonellosis	la salmonelosis
stomatitis	la estomatitis
traumatic reticuloperitonitis (hardware disease)	la reticuloperitonitis traumática *or* la gastritis traumática

The eye, ear, and skin [*El ojo, el oído y la piel*]

alopecia	la alopecia
bovine ocular squamous cell carcinoma	el carcinoma ocular bovino de las células escamosas

conjunctivitis	la conjuntivitis
deafness	la sordera
dermatitis	la dermatitis
dermatophytosis	la dermatofitosis
horn fly	la mosca del cuerno
infectious kerato-conjunctivitis	la queratoconjuntivitis infecciosa
keratitis	la queratitis
mange	la sarna
papillomatosis	la papilomatosis
parakeratosis	la paraqueratosis
pediculosis	la pediculosis
pseudo-cowpox	la pseudo-viruela bovina
tick infestation	la infestación por garrapatas
stable flies	las moscas de establo

The immune system [*El sistema inmune*]

allergy	la alergía
anaphylactic shock	el shock anafiláctico

Metabolic and production-related diseases
[*Las enfermedades metabólicas y relacionadas a la producción*]

fat cow syndrome	el síndrome de la vaca gorda
hypomagnesemic tetany	la tetania hipomagnesémica
ketosis	la acetonemia
obesity	la obesidad
parturient paresis	la fiebre de leche

The musculoskeletal system [*El sistema musculoesquelético*]

arthritis	la artritis
contracted flexor tendons	los tendones flexores contraídos
dislocation	la dislocación
foreign body penetration of the sole	la penetración de la suela por cuerpo extraño
fracture	la fractura
lameness	la cojera
pododermatitis	la pododermatitis
osteitis	la osteítis
sarcocystosis	la sarcocistosis

The nervous system [*El sistema nervioso*]

Haemophilus septicemia of cattle	la septicemia del ganado por hemófilus
meningitis	la meningitis
neoplasia	la neoplasia
rabies	la rabia
tick paralysis	la parálisis por garrapatas

Physical influences [*Las influencias físicas*]

burns	las quemaduras
electric shock	el shock eléctrico
electrocution by lightning strike	el electrocutamiento por tormenta eléctrica
frostbite	la quemadura por frío
high mountain disease	la enfermedad de las alturas
hyperthermia	la hipertermia
hypothermia	la hipotermia
motion sickness	el mareo
thoracic trauma	el trauma torácico
wounds	las heridas

The reproductive system [*El sistema reproductivo*]

abortion	el aborto
agalactia	la agalactia
balanopostitis	la balanopostitis
bovine genital campylobacteriosis	la campilobacteriosis genital bovina
bovine trichomoniases	la tricomoníasis bovina
brucellosis	la brucelosis
dystocia	la distocia
epididymitis	la epididimitis
infertility	la infertilidad
mastitis	la mastitis
metritis	la metritis
orchitis	la orquitis
ovarian cyst	el quiste ovárico
pyometra	la piometra
retained placenta	la retención de placenta
uterine prolapse	el prolapso uterino
vaginal prolapse	el prolapso vaginal

vaginitis	la vaginitis
vulvitis	la vulvitis

The respiratory system [*El sistema respiratorio*]

acute bovine pulmonary emphysema and edema	el enfisema y el edema pulmonar agudo bovino
aspiration pneumonia	la neumonía por aspiración
bovine pneumonic pasteurellosis	la pasteurelosis neumónica bovina
bovine respiratory disease complex	el complejo respiratorio bovino
calf diphtheria	la difteria de los terneros
endemic pneumonia in calves	la neumonía endémica de los terneros
infectious bovine rhinotracheitis	la rinotraqueítis infecciosa bovina
laryngeal edema	el edema laríngeo
laryngitis	la laringitis
lungworm infection	la infección por gusanos pulmonares
pharyngitis	la faringitis
pulmonary emphysema	el enfisema pulmonar

The urinary system [*El sistema urinario*]

acute renal failure	la falla renal aguda
bovine cystitis and pyelonephritis	la cistitis y la pielonefritis bovina
chronic renal failure	la falla renal crónica
hematuria	la hematuria
nephrotic syndrome	el síndrome nefrótico
polyuria	la poliuria
proteinuria	la proteinuria
renal tubular defects	los defectos de los túbulos renales
urinary obstruction	la obstrucción urinaria
urinary tract infection	la infección del tracto urinario

Generalized conditions [*Las condiciones generalizadas*]

actinobacillosis	la actinobacilosis
actinomycosis	la actinomicosis
anthrax	el ántrax
aspergillosis	la aspergilosis

bacillary hemoglobinuria	la hemoglobinuria bacilar
black leg	la pierna negra
candidosis	la candidíasis
dehydration	la deshidratación
enterotoxemia	la enterotoxemia
leptospirosis	la leptospirosis
listeriosis	la listeriosis
malignant catarral fever	la fiebre catarral maligna
malignant edema	el edema maligno
paratuberculosis	la paratuberculosis
shock	el shock
tuberculosis	la tuberculosis

CHAPTER 11

Horses

Equestrianism is an ancient tradition in Hispanic culture, and indeed most of our Anglo customs and terms stem from Hispanic roots. What we assume is English is often warped Spanish, as you can see in these terms:

lasso	el lazo
buckaroo	el vaquero
cinch	la cincha
mustang	el mustang
corral	el corral
riata	la reata
roan	ruano

In Hispanic countries, it is not unusual to remember the names of important people's horses as well as the human names; the hero El Cid rode Babieca, and the stringy Don Quixote rode the equally bony Rocinante (a play on *rocín,* a nag). Horses were so important to Spaniards that the *conquistadores* included their numbers and names in their histories; for instance, see Bernal Díaz's *True History of the Conquest of New Spain,* in which he accounts for the fate of every horse in the expedition. After all, the term for "gentleman" is *caballero,* a mounted man. An ordinary soldier, on the other hand, is a *peón,* literally a foot (*pie*) soldier; the same word gave us "pawn," the cannon fodder in chess. For their part, the Aztecs held the Spanish horses in such esteem that they sacrificed them alongside human captives, and placed their heads on the skull racks in the main plaza. Even today, a peasant who owns a horse considers himself superior to his neighbors who do not, and the wealthy classes still include gorgeous horses as essential symbols of prestige.

> **Important note:** conditions already covered in the chapter on cattle, such as anemia, are not repeated here.

Special Vocabulary

Special vocabulary for horses
[*El vocabulario especial de los caballos*]

stallion	el semental, el garañón
mare	la yegua
foal	el potrillo, la potranquita
colt	el potro
filly	la potranca
gelding	el caballo castrado
donkey	el burro
mule	la mula
stall	la caballeriza
to foal	parir
to neigh	relinchar
to trot	trotar
to rasp	escofinar
horse shoeing	el herraje
horseshoe	la herradura

Illnesses

The blood, lymphatic, and cardiovascular system
[*El sistema sanguíneo, linfático y cardiovascular*]

aneurysm	el aneurisma
embolism	el embolismo
equine infectious anemia	la anemia infecciosa equina
hemolytic disease of newborn foals	la enfermedad hemolítica de potros recién nacidos
lymphangitis	la linfangitis
thrombosis	la trombosis

The digestive system [*El sistema digestivo*]

choke	la obstrucción del esófago
colic	el cólico
colitis-x	la colitis-equis
dilation of the esophagus	el megaesófago

esophageal diverticulum	el divertículo esofágico
gastritis	la gastritis

The endocrine system [*El sistema endocrino*]

diabetes mellitus	la diabetes mellitus
hirsutism	el hirsutismo
hypoadrenocorticism	el hipoadrenocorticismo
pituitary tumor	el tumor pituitario

Eye, ear, and skin [*El ojo, el oído y la piel*]

cataract	la catarata
hives, urticaria	la urticaria
pyoderma	la pioderma
sweet itch in horses	la hipersensibilidad a culicoides

The immune system [*El sistema inmune*]

anterior uveitis	la uveítis anterior
autoimmune hemolytic anemia	la anemia hemolítica autoinmune

The musculoskeletal system [*El sistema musculoesquelético*]

azoturia	la azoturia
bursitis	la bursitis

The nervous system [*El sistema nervioso*]

equine encephalomyelitis	la encefalomielitis equina
facial paralysis	la parálisis facial
tetanus	el tétanos
tremors	los temblores, los tremores

The respiratory system [*El sistema respiratorio*]

chronic obstructive pulmonary disease	la enfermedad pulmonar crónica obstructiva
equine influenza	la influenza equina
equine viral rhinopneumonitis	la rinoneumonitis viral equina
laryngeal hemiplegia	la hemiplejia laríngea
pleurisy	la pleuresía
strangles	el distemper equino; la papera equina

The urinary system [*El sistema urinario*]

uroperitoneum in foals	el uroperitoneo en potros

Generalized conditions [*Las condiciones generalizadas*]

blastomycosis	la blastomicosis
equine monocytic ehrlichiosis	la erliquiosis monocítica equina
equine viral arteritis	la arteritis viral equina
septicemia in foals	la septicemia de los potros

12

Sheep and Goats

Spain was once a center for woolen cloth (before the new cotton fabrics became the preferred underclothing material—ouch!), and enormous herds of sheep and goats moved from pasture to pasture. The law gave preference to these herds over other animal herds and certainly over human property. No one could put up fences that would obstruct the sheep's path. Sheep and goats don't enjoy that kind of privilege today, but they are still very common throughout the Hispanic world. A favorite barbeque meat is kid, and it is very well prepared indeed. Many cheeses are made from sheep or goat's milk rather than cow's milk.

Important note: Conditions already covered in the previous two chapters are not repeated here.

Special Vocabulary

Special vocabulary for sheep and goats
[*El vocabulario especial de las ovejas y las cabras*]

ewe	la oveja hembra
ram (sheep)	el carnero
lamb	el cordero, la cordera
buck	el macho cabrío
doe	la cabra hembra
kid	el cabrito, la cabrita
flock	el rebaño
docking	el descolado
to dock	descolar
to milk	ordeñar

to bleat	balar
teat dipping	el enjuage de los pezones
disbudding	el descornado

Illnesses

The blood, lymphatic, and cardiovascular system
[*El sistema sanguíneo, linfático y cardiovascular*]

caseous lymphadenitis	la linfadenitis caseosa

The digestive system [*El sistema digestivo*]

enterotoxemia	la enterotoxemia
indigestion	la indigestión
intestinal obstruction	la obstrucción intestinal

Eye, ear, and skin [*El ojo, el oído y la piel*]

contagious ecthyma	el ectima contagioso
dermatophilosis	la dermatofilosis
sheep ked	la infestación por *Melophagus ovinus*
ulcerative dermatosis in sheep	la dermatosis ulcerativa de las ovejas

Metabolic and production-related diseases
[*Las enfermedades metabólicas y relacionadas a la producción*]

hypomagnesemic tetany	la tetania hipomagnesémica

The musculoskeletal system [*El sistema musculoesquéletico*]

foot abscess	el abceso en la pata
ovine interdigital dermatitis	la dermatitis ovina interdigital
white muscle disease	la enfermedad del músculo blanco

The nervous system [*El sistema nervioso*]

enzootic ataxia	la ataxia enzoótica
scrapie	el scrapie

The reproductive system [*El sistema reproductivo*]

chlamydial abortion of ewes	el aborto clamidial de las ovejas
epididymitis of rams	la epididimitis de los carneros
ovine genital campylo-bacteriosis	la campilobacteriosis genital ovina

The respiratory system [*El sistema respiratorio*]

contagious caprine pleuropneumonia	la pleuroneumonía contagiosa caprina
nonprogressive pneumonia in sheep	la neumonía atípica de las ovejas
progressive pneumonia in sheep	la neumonía progresiva de las ovejas
pulmonary adenomatosis	la adenomatosis pulmonar
sheep nose bot	la infestación por oestrus ovis

The urinary system [*El sistema urinario*]

urolithiasis	la urolitiásis

Generalized conditions [*Las condiciones generalizadas*]

caprine arthritis	la artritis caprina
caprine encephalitis	la encefalitis caprina
septicemic pasteurellosis of sheep	la pasteurelosis septicémica de las ovejas
toxoplasmosis	la toxoplasmosis

CHAPTER 13

Swine

When Spain was divided culturally between the Christians, the Moors, and the Jews, the Christians began the custom of eating pork on Friday evenings to differentiate themselves from the other religions. Nowadays, the reason for that custom has long disappeared, but it is still common for certain traditional pork dishes to be eaten on weekends. (Similarly, the custom of having clam chowder as the soup of the day on Fridays in U.S. restaurants stems from the Catholic prohibition on eating meat on Fridays.) Today in poor Latin American countries, it is more common to eat pork than beef because swine are more adaptable to climate and diet, reproduce more rapidly, and need less land than cattle. Poor families use every scrap of a pig, wasting nothing; the ears, for example, are often stewed with beans. In the wealthier countries, such as Argentina, fine beef is eaten in astounding quantities, and pork is more likely to show up in sausages. Suckling pigs are a common Christmas or special occasion dish, however.

> **Important note:** Conditions already covered in the previous three chapters are not repeated here.

Special Vocabulary

Special vocabulary for swine [*El vocabulario especial de los cerdos*]

boar	el verraco
sow	la cerda, el vientre
piglet	el lechón
gilt	la cerda de remplazo
barrow	el cerdo castrado
weaned swine	el cerdo destetado

growing swine	el cerdo en crecimiento
finishing swine	el cerdo en finalización
pork	el puerco
iron shot	la inyección de hierro
clipping of the needle teeth	el descolmillado
ear marking, ear notching	el muesqueo
farrowing	el parto
pig snare	la asa trompas

Illnesses

The blood, lymphatic, and cardiovascular system [*El sistema sanguíneo, linfático y cardiovascular*]

| hemolytic disease of newborn pigs | la enfermedad hemolítica de los cerdos recién nacidos |
| streptococcal lymphadenitis of swine | la linfadenitis por estreptococos |

The digestive system [*El sistema digestivo*]

enteric colibacillosis	la colibacilosis entérica
parasitosis by	la infestación por
Ascaris suum	la ascariosis
Strongyloides ransomi	la estrongiloidosis
Trichuris suis	la trichuriosis
rotoviral enteritis	la enteritis por rotavirus
swine dysentery	la disentería porcina
transmissible gastroenteritis	la gastroenteritis transmisible

Eye, ear, and skin [*El ojo, el oído y la piel*]

| exudative epidermitis | la epidermitis exudativa |
| necrotic ear syndrome | el síndrome del oído necrótico |

Metabolic and production-related diseases [*Las enfermedades metabólicas y relacionadas a la producción*]

| hypoglicemia of piglets | la hipoglicemia de los lechones |
| malignant hyperthermia | la hipertermia maligna |

The musculoskeletal system [*El sistema musculoesquelético*]

| splay legs | la hipoplasia miofibrilar |

The nervous system [*El sistema nervioso*]

arsanilic acid poisoning	el envenenamiento por ácido arsanílico
coronaviral encephalomyelitis	la encefalomielitis por coronavirus
edema disease	la enfermedad del edema
porcine enteroviral encephalomyelitis	la encefalomielitis por enterovirus porcino
pseudorabies	la seudorabia

The reproductive system [*El sistema reproductivo*]

porcine reproductive and respiratory syndrome	el síndrome respiratorio y reproductivo porcino

The urinary system [*El sistema urinario*]

porcine cystitis	la cistitis porcina

Generalized conditions [*Las condiciones generalizadas*]

erysipelas	la erisipela
Glässer's disease	la poliserositis porcina
porcine streptococcal infection	la infección por estreptococos
trichinosis	la triquinelosis
toxoplasmosis	la toxoplasmosis

CHAPTER 14

Dogs and Cats

For many U.S. veterinarians, dogs and cats make up the bulk of their practice. In Hispanic America, however, vets mainly see large animals because they have such vital economic importance. Yet Hispanic Americans do love their dogs and cats, and commercial products for them are increasingly generating revenues. Vets specializing in small animals—though still few in number in comparison with the United States—are becoming more common in cities. Certain breeds of dogs are native to the Americas, and their special place in pre-Columbian society is reflected in the sensitive pottery images found among the Maya and Aztecs. Dogs were food animals in those days despite the fact that certain breeds had the charming attribute of not barking.

Important note: Conditions already covered in the previous four chapters are not repeated here.

Special Vocabulary

Special vocabulary for small animals
[El vocabulario especial de las pequeñas especies]

pet	la mascota
pet owner	el dueño, la dueña
male cat	el gato macho, el gato
female cat	el gato hembra, la gata
kitten	el gatito, la gatita
neutered male cat	el gato macho capado

spayed female cat	la gata esterilizada, castrada; la gata ovariohisterectomizada
male dog	el perro macho
bitch	la perra
puppy	el cachorrito, la cachorrita; el perrito, la perrita
neutered male dog	el perro macho capado
spayed female dog	la perra esterilizada, castrada; la perra overiohisterectomizada
to bark	ladrar
to meow	maullar
to purr	ronronear
to whine	lloriquear
to bite	morder (ue)
to scratch (to draw blood)	arañar
to scratch (an itch)	rasgar
litter	la camada
kennel	la perrera
collar	el collar
leash	la correa
ID tag	la placa de identificación
carrier	el transportín
toys	los juguetes
catnip	la menta de los gatos
litter box, litter tray	la bandeja de arena
kitty litter	la arena
scratching post	el rascador
grooming	el aseo
ear cleaning	la limpieza de oídos
anal gland grooming	el aseo de glándulas anales
nail clipping	el corte de uñas
antiflea treatment	el tratamiento antipulgas
comb; to comb	el peine; peinar
metal-toothed comb	el peine de púas metálicas
brush; to brush	el cepillo; cepillar
bristle brush	el cepillo de cerdas finas
shampoo	el champú
bath; to bathe	el baño; bañar
food bowl	el comedero
water bowl	el bebedero

food (for animals)	el pienso
dry food	la comida seca
wet food	la comida húmeda
canned food	la comida enlatada
brand (of food)	la marca
boarding (at a kennel)	la pensión

Illnesses

The blood, lymphatic, and cardiovascular system *[El sistema sanguíneo, linfático y cardiovascular]*

canine heartworm infection	la dirofilariásis
canine malignant lymphoma	el linfoma maligno canino
feline infectious anemia	la anemia infecciosa felina
feline lymphosarcoma	el linfosarcoma felino
feline leukemia	la leucemia felina
hemolytic disease of newborn puppies and kittens	la enfermedad hemolítica de perros y gatos recién nacidos
polyarteritis	la poliarteritis
polycythemia	la policitemia
vasculitis	la vasculitis

The digestive system *[El sistema digestivo]*

fur ball	la bola de pelo
cough up a fur ball	vomitar la bola de pelo
anal sac disease	la enfermedad del saco anal
canine coronaviral	la gastroenteritis canina; gastroenteritis por coronavirus
canine oral papillomatosis	la papilomatosis oral canina
dental caries	las caries dentales
esophageal stenosis	la estenosis esofágica
exocrine disease of the pancreas	la enfermedad del pancreas exócrino
gastric dilation-volvulus	la dilatación gástrica-vólvulo
gastric foreign body	el cuerpo extraño gástrico
giardiasis	la giardiasis
gingivitis	la gingivitis
malabsorption syndrome	el síndrome de mala absorción
mouth burns	las quemaduras bocales

| sialadenitis | la sialadenisis |
| small intestinal obstruction | la obstrucción del intestino delgado |

The endocrine system *[El sistema endocrino]*

pancreitis	la pancreatitis
hyperadrenocorticism	el hiperadrenocorticismo
hyperthyroidism	el hipertiroidismo
hypothryoidism	el hipotiroidismo

Eye, ear, and skin *[El ojo, el oído, y la piel]*

fleas	las pulgas
ticks	las garrapatas
acantosis	la acantosis
alopecia	la alopecia
eczema nasi of dogs	la dermatitis nasal canina
flea allergy dermatitis	la dermatitis por alergia a pulgas
flea infestation	la infestación por pulgas
glaucoma	el glaucoma
interdigital cyst	el quiste interdigital
otitis	la otitis
prolapse of the eye	el prolapso ocular

The immune system *[El sistema inmune]*

| autoimmune thyroiditis | la tiroiditis autoinmune |
| systemic lupus erythematous | el lupus eritematoso sistémico |

The musculoskeletal system *[El sistema musculoesquelético]*

diaphragmatic hernia	la hernia diafragmática
canine hip dysplasia	la displasia de cadera
hyperparathyroidism	el hiperparatiroidismo
hypoparathyroidism	el hipoparatiroidismo
Lyme disease	la borreliosis
osteitis	la osteítis
osteoarthritis	la osteoartritis
spondylosis deformans	la spondilosis deformante

The nervous system *[El sistema nervioso]*

| epilepsy | la epilepsia |
| intervertebral disk disease | la enfermedad del disco intervertebral |

seizures	las convulsiones
spinal trauma	el trauma espinal

Physical influences *[Las influencias físicas]*

accidents caused by . . .	los accidentes causados por . . .
automobiles	los automóviles, los autos
other animals	los otros animales
sharp objects	los objetos punzocortantes
gun shots	los disparos
blunt impact	el golpe
falling	la caída
drowning	el ahogamiento
poisoning	el envenenamiento

The reproductive system *[El sistema reproductivo]*

mammary tumor	el tumor mamario
prostatitis	la prostatitis
pseudopregnancy	la seudopreñez
spaying, ovariohysterectomy	la ovariohisterectomía
transmissible canine venereal tumor	el tumor venéreo transmisible

The respiratory system *[El sistema respiratorio]*

kennel cough	la tos de las perreras
feline respiratory disease complex	el complejo respiratorio felino
infectious tracheobronchitis of dogs	la traqueobronquitis infecciosa canina
lung flukes	los tremátodos pulmonares
rhinitis and sinusitis	la rinitis y la sinusitis
tonsillitis	la tonsilitis

The urinary system *[El sistema urinario]*

canine urolithiasis	la urolitiasis canina
feline urological syndrome	el síndrome urológico felino
tumors of the kidney	los tumores renales

Generalized conditions *[Las condiciones generalizadas]*

canine distemper	el moquillo; el distémper canino
canine erlichiosis	la erliquiosis canina

canine herpesviral infection	la infección por herpesvirus canino
canine parvoviral infection	la infección por parvovirus canino
coccidioidomycosis	la coccidioidomicosis
cryptococcosis	la criptococosis
feline infectious peritonitis	la peritonitis infecciosa felina
feline panleukopenia	la panleucopenia felina
histoplasmosis	la histoplasmosis
infectious canine hepatitis	la hepatitis infecciosa canina
Rocky Mountain spotted fever	la fiebre de las Montañas Rocallosas
salmon poisoning disease	la enfermedad por salmón contaminado; la intoxicación por salmón

CHAPTER 15

Exotic Pets

These days, a veterinarian's waiting room may resemble a zoo. Alongside your clients with their traditional dogs and cats, some may be holding cages with snakes, geckos, or toucans. Keeping reptiles and rodents as pets is still new in the Spanish-speaking world, but it has long been the custom to keep birds. Balconies and interior courtyards are frequently adorned with cages of pampered avian pets. In Andean countries, guinea pigs are numerous—as food animals. Mmm, tasty!

> **Important note:** Conditions already covered in the previous five chapters are not repeated here.

Special Vocabulary

There are two words in Spanish for "bird."

- *el pájaro, los pájaros*—this term comes from ordinary speech.
- *el ave, las aves*—this term is a little more formal and scientific sounding.

To specify that the animal is an adult male, add *macho* after the noun: *la tortuga macho; el loro macho.*

To specify that the animal is an adult female, add *hembra* after the noun: *la tortuga hembra; el loro hembra.*

"Offspring" is *la cría: la cría de hamster.*

Birds *[Las aves]*

parakeet	el perico, el periquito
canary	el canario

lovebird	el agapornis, el lorito del amor, los inseparables
dove, pigeon	la paloma
cockatoo	la cacatúa
cockatiel, quarrion	la ninfa, la carolina
conure	el loro
parrot	la cotorra, el loro
macaw	la guacamaya
toucan	el tucán
falcon	el halcón
kestrel	el halconcillo
ostrich	el avestruz
emu	el emú
baby birds	los polluelos

Rodents [Los roedores]

ferret	el hurón
chinchilla	la chinchilla
rabbit	el conejo
hamster	el hamster
guinea pig	la cobaya; el cuyo; el conejillo de Indias; el cuy
gerbil	el jerbo
rat	la rata
mouse	el ratón

Reptiles [Los reptiles]

snake	la víbora, la serpiente
grass snake, water snake	la culebra
python	el pitón
boa	la boa
rat snake	la ratonera
iguana	la iguana
monitor lizard	el varano
gecko	el geco
lizard	la lagartija
anole	el anoli
chameleon	el camaleón
turtle	la tortuga
tortoise	la tortuga terrestre
box turtle	la tortuga de caja

Amphibians *[Los anfibios]*
frog	la rana
toad	el sapo
salamander	la salamandra, el tritón
axolotl	el axolote

Invertebrates *[Los invertebrados]*
scorpion	el escorpión
tarantula	la tarántula

Body Parts *[Las partes corporales]*
beak	el pico
crest	la cresta
crop	el buche
feather	la pluma
foot	la pata
fur	el pelo
gizzard	la molleja
nail	la uña
plumage	el plumaje
shell, tortoise shell	el caparazón
tail	la cola
talon	la garra
wing, wings	el ala, las alas

Nutrition, Feeding *[La nutrición, la alimentación]*
banana	el plátano
birdseed	el alpiste
biscuit, cookie	la galleta
broccoli	el brécol
chew bar	la barrita de pienso
cricket	el grillo
cucumber	el pepino
cuttle bone	el hueso de jibia; el escudo de sepia
dry food	la comida seca; las croquetas
flaxseed	el lino; la semilla de lino
fruit	la fruta
grit	el grit
hemp seed	la semilla de cáñamo

insects	los insectos
lettuce	la lechuga
live food	el alimento vivo
mealworm	el tenebrio; el gusano de la harina
millet	el panizo; el mijo
nectar	el néctar
orange	la naranja
pellets	las bolitas
rapeseed	la semilla de colza
red mosquito larva	la larva roja de mosquito
seeds	las semillas
spinach	la espinaca
sunflower seeds	la pipa; la pipa de girasol
tomato	el tomate
treat	la golosina
vegetables; fresh vegetables	las verduras; las verduras frescas

Housing [El alojamiento]

aviary	el aviario; la pajarera
bars; metal bars	las rejas; la rejilla metálica
bath; bathing pool	la bañera
cage	la jaula
dovecot, pigeon loft	el palomar
exercise wheel	la rueda de ejercicio
food dish	el recipiente
hideaway; retreat	el cobijo
perch	la percha
swing	el columpio
tank	el tanque
terrarium	el terrario
water bottle	la botella de agua
water bowl	el bebedero
wood shavings	la viruta de madera

Behavior [El comportamiento]

beat, flap its wings	batir las alas
diurnal	diurno, diurna; de día
feather picking	el picoteo de pluma
lay eggs	poner huevos

lower (the crest)	retraer
raise (the crest)	alzar
nest	el nido (noun); anidar (verb)
nocturnal	nocturno, nocturna; de noche
pick its feathers	picarse las plumas
preen	arreglarse las plumas con el pico

Illnesses and Conditions *[Las enfermedades y las condiciones]*

asthma	el asma
cold; catarrh	el catarro
diphtheria	la difteria
eye infection	la infección ocular; la infección del ojo
eye swelling	el hinchazón de ojos
fungus	los hongos
itching	la picazón
lack of vitamin C	la carencia de vitamina C; la falta de vitamina C
lice; bird lice	el piojo; el piojillo
mite	el ácaro
molting	la muda
nail clip	el corte de uñas
pathological molting	la muda patológica
permanent molting	la muda permanente
psitacosis	la psitacosis
salmonella	la salmonelosis
shell-less eggs	los huevos sin cáscara
shut eyes	los ojos cerrados
swollen eyes	los ojos hinchados
inactive; lethargic	inactivo, inactiva; letárgico, letárgica
softening of the shell	el reblandecimiento del caparazón
uninterested in eating	sin ganas de comer
vitamin deficiency	la avitaminosis
wing clip	el corte de alas
worms	las lombrices; los gusanos

Registration Forms

Information about the Owners [*Datos sobre los dueños*] ____

Owner	el dueño, la dueña
Name	nombre
First name	nombre; nombre de pila
Last name	apellido(s) (See cultural note in Chapter 2.)
Middle initial	inicial del segundo nombre
Address	dirección
Street	calle
Apartment number	número de apartamento
Apt. no.	núm. apto.
City	ciudad
State	estado
Zip code	código postal
Phone (home)	teléfono (casa)
Phone (work)	teléfono (empleo)
Phone (cell)	teléfono (celular)
E-mail	correo electrónico
May we call you at work?	¿Nos permite llamarle a su empleo?
Yes ____ **no** ____	Sí ____ No ____
In case of emergency, call . . .	En caso de emergencia, llame . . .
How did you hear about us? (If most of your clients are of Mexican heritage)	¿Cómo se enteró de nosotros?

How did you hear about us? (If most of your clients are of other Spanish-speaking heritages)	¿Cómo supo de nosotros?
payment method	método de pagar
cash	efectivo
credit	crédito
credit card	tarjeta de crédito
debit	débito
debit card	tarjeta de débito
expiration date	fecha de vencimiento
check	cheque
driver's license number	el número de la licencia de conducir
social security number	el número de la seguridad social
signature	firma
date	fecha
Please give picture ID to the receptionist.	Favor de darle a la recepcionista un documento de identidad con foto.

Note: The legal authorization for treatment and other legal agreements should be translated by licensed legal translators. See the business pages of your phone book.

Pet Information *[Datos sobre la mascota]*

pet name	nombre de la mascota
dog/cat/other	perro/gato/otro
breed	raza
color and markings	color y manchas
male/female	macho/hembra
altered	capado/capada
birthday	fecha de nacimiento
age	edad
date of last vaccinations	fecha de las últimas vacunas
pet's daily diet	dieta diaria de la mascota
brand of food	marca de la alimentación
frequency of meals	frecuencia de alimentación
once a day	una vez al día
twice a day	dos veces al día

food out all the time	siempre disponible
daily vitamins	vitaminas diarias
medication(s)	medicamento(s)
name of medication	nombre del medicamento
dose	dósis
times a day	veces al día
allergies or reactions	alergias o reacciones
hours spent outside each day	horas pasadas afuera cada día

Boarding *[La pensión]*

collar, leash, carrier	collar, correa, transportín
toys	juguetes
personal belongings	efectos personales
We are not responsible for lost or damaged items.	No somos responsables por los efectos perdidos o dañados.
proof of current vaccinations	prueba de las vacunas actuales
We require that the pet not have external parasites (such as fleas, lice, mites).	Se requiere que la mascota no tenga los parásitos externos (como las garrapatas, los piojos, los ácaros).

Requested Services *[Servicios solicitados]*

physical exam	examen físico
vaccinations	inoculación
flea treatment	tratamiento antipulgas
flea shampoo	champú antipulgas
bath	baño
ear cleaning	limpieza de oídos
nail trim	corte de uñas
anal gland cleaning	aseo de glándulas anales

Answer Key to Exercises

EXERCISE 1-2

el toro, los toros
la vaca, las vacas
el caballo, los caballos
la yegua, las yeguas
el gallo, los gallos
la gallina, las gallinas
el perro, los perros
la perra, las perras
el gato, los gatos
la gata, las gatas
el macho cabrío, los machos cabríos
la cabra, las cabras
el carnero, los carneros
la oveja, las ovejas
el cerdo, los cerdos
la cerda, las cerdas
el pato, los patos
la pata, las patas
el conejo, los conejos
la coneja, las conejas

EXERCISE 1-3

el toro, un toro
la vaca, una vaca
el caballo, un caballo
la yegua, una yegua
etc.

EXERCISE 1-5

el antípole, los antípoles
el oso, los osos

el camello, los camellos
el cocodrilo, los cocodrilos
el venado, el ciervo, los venados, los ciervos
el elefante, los elefantes
el pez, los peces [The z changes to c before
    e, but the sound doesn't change.]
el zorro, los zorros
la jirafa, las jirafas
etc.

EXERCISE 1-6

el hipopótamo, un hipopótamo
el león, un león
la llama, una llama
el mono, un mono
el avestruz, un avestruz
el rinoceronte, un rinoceronte
etc.

EXERCISE 2-1

1. el caballo blanco, la gata blanca, los
   cerdos blancos
2. la pata lastimada, las piernas
   lastimadas, los pies lastimados, el ojo
   lastimado
3. el perro enfermo, las cebras enfermas,
   los cabritos enfermos, la oveja enferma
4. cinco pulgas, cinco tumores, cinco días
5. muchos animales, muchas infecciones,
   mucha sangre, mucho olor
6. la orina sanguinolenta, las heces
   sanguinolentas, el moco sanguinolento,
   el vómito sanguinolento

7. el diagnóstico posible, los problemas posibles, la solución posible, las terapias posibles
8. una enfermedad respiratoria, un ruido respiratorio, los problemas respiratorios, los exámenes respiratorios

EXERCISE 2-2

1. la gata anémica
2. las convulsiones frecuentes
3. el cerdo letárgico
4. los quistes pequeños
5. las fiebres repentinas
6. las costillas lastimadas
7. el parto dificultoso
8. poca energía
9. los perros capados
10. la dificultad respiratoria

EXERCISE 2-3

1. el abdomen distendido
2. los ojos llorosos
3. la almohadilla infectada
4. el corazón irregular
5. la vulva sanguinolenta
6. la boca seca
7. los perros recién nacidos
8. los pulmones congestionados
9. el ano impactado
10. las tripas equinas

EXERCISE 2-4

1. las rodillas
2. el hocico
3. la cabra
4. el problema (Watch for this one! It's a Greek word!)
5. la sangre
6. la mastitis
7. la fiebre
8. los cuernos
9. la cruz
10. la ubre
11. las gatas
12. las enfermedades
13. los osos
14. el pez

15. las plumas
16. el sorgo
17. las vitaminas
18. los suplementos
19. el tórax
20. el síntoma (Another Greek one!)
21. el moquillo
22. la diarrea
23. las llamas
24. el animal
25. la uña
26. las infecciones
27. la pata
28. el ojo

EXERCISE 3-1

1. yo vendo, tú vendas, él/ella/usted venda, nosotros vendamos, ellos/ellas/ustedes vendan
2. reviso, revisas, revisa, revisamos, revisan
3. inoculo, inoculas, inocula, inoculamos, inoculan
4. comprendo, comprendes, comprende, comprendemos, comprenden
5. debo, debes, debe, debemos, deben
6. creo, crees, cree, creemos, creen
7. añado, añades, añade, añadimos, añaden
8. recibo, recibes, recibe, recibimos, reciben
9. sufro, sufres, sufre, sufrimos, sufren
10. ordeño, ordeñas, ordeña, ordeñamos, ordeñan

EXERCISE 3-2

1. la cerda pare, las cerdas paren
2. el gato lame, los gatos lamen
3. el problema ocurre, los problemas ocurren
4. el perrito tose, los perritos tosen
5. la yegua respira, las yeguas respiran
6. el perro jadea, los perros jadean
7. el loro come, los loros comen
8. la oveja padece de, las ovejas padecen de
9. la herida parece, las heridas parecen
10. la llama cojea, las llamas cojean

EXERCISE 3-3
1. padece
2. tose
3. late
4. revisamos
5. venda
6. creo
7. parecen
8. limpian
9. debe
10. beben, comen

EXERCISE 3-4
1. yo recomiendo, tú recomiendas, él/ella/usted recomienda, nosotros recomendamos, ellos/ellas/ustedes recomiendan
2. quiero, quieres, quiere, queremos, quieren
3. sugiero, sugieres, sugiere, sugerimos, sugieren
4. pierdo, pierdes, pierde, perdemos, pierden
5. tiemblo, tiemblas, tiembla, temblamos, tiemblan
6. pruebo, pruebas, prueba, probamos, prueban
7. puedo, puedes, puede, podemos, pueden
8. vuelvo, vuelves, vuelve, volvemos, vuelven
9. sigo, sigues, sigue, seguimos, siguen
10. pido, pides, pide, pedimos, piden

EXERCISE 3-5
1. cuesta, cuestan
2. vuela, vuelan
3. muerde, muerden
4. previene, previenen
5. huele, huelen
6. muestra, muestran

EXERCISE 3-6
1. tiembla
2. vuelven
3. recomiendo
4. queremos

5. puede
6. prueban
7. cuesta
8. sigue
9. pierden
10. recomendamos
11. pide

EXERCISE 4-1
1. está
2. tienen
3. es
4. tiene
5. va
6. está, tiene
7. tienen
8. es
9. está, va
10. están, tienen, están

EXERCISE 4-2
1. El caballo tiene cólico. Tiene dolor y está grave.
2. El gato tiene fiebre y los ojos están hundidos.
3. Voy a hacer unas pruebas. Entonces voy a consultar con un especialista or una especialista.
4. ¡Spot está mejor! La temperatura está normal.
5. La vaca está gestante, pero está débil y un poco flaca.
6. Los perros tienen moquillo. Están muy enfermos.
7. La lesión está mejor, pero todavía está un poco inflamada.
8. La ternera tiene dificultad para respirar, y la mucosidad está verde.
9. El señor González es el dueño de una lechería moderna. Es un cliente estimado. Es muy inteligente y simpático también. Voy a examinar sus vacas mañana.
10. Pooky no está grave. Tiene parásitos, pero esta pastilla va a eliminar/expulsar los parásitos. En una semana, va a estar bien.

11. Voy a vendar la herida y recetar unas pastillas.
12. La especialista/el especialista va a revisar los resultados de la prueba y recomendar un tratamiento.

EXERCISE 4-3

Notice that there are several ways to describe these illnesses. Here are some suggestions.

1. El carnero no quiere comer, tiene dificultad para marchar, está flaco, las heces están infrecuentes y escasas, tiene fiebre, tiene dificultad para respirar, tiene dolor, el abdomen está duro o distentido, etc.
2. El cerdo tiene dificultad para respirar, tiene fiebre, tiene tos persistente, tiene tos seca, etc.
3. La gata no quiere comer, está débil, tiene orina escasa o ausente, tiene temblores, marcha con dificultad, pierde peso, etc.
4. El caballo tiene dolor abdominal, no quiere comer, trata de beber pero no puede, marcha mucho, las heces están impactadas, tiene shock, tiene dificultad para respirar, no hay ruidos en el abdomen, etc.
5. La vaca tiene disminución de la leche, tione dolor en el pezón, los pezones están inflamados, la leche está acuosa o no normal, hay masas o lesiones o abcesos en la ubre, tiene edema en la ubre, etc.

EXERCISE 4-4

1. Este medicamento va a curar el problema.
   Este medicamento debe curar el problema.
   Este medicamento puede curar el problema.
2. Podemos volver mañana.
   Tenemos que volver mañana.
   Vamos a volver mañana.

3. Voy a tomar unos rayos x.
   Necesito tomar unos rayos x.
   Acabo de tomar unos rayos x.
   Tengo que tomar unos rayos x.

EXERCISE 4-5

1. Hay un problema.
2. Hay cinco vacas con brucelosis.
3. Hay sangre en la orina.
4. No hay signos de leucemia.
5. Hay un medicamento nuevo para esta condición.

EXERCISE 5-1

1. Hace un día que el caballo sufre de cólico. *Or* Hace un día.
2. Hace unos pocos días que la orina está sanguinolenta.
3. Hace una semana que la gata tiene la lesión.
4. Hace tres días que el toro no come.
5. Hace doce horas que la oveja trata de parir.
6. Hace dos semanas que el canario tiene parásitos.
7. Hace un mes, más o menos, que tiene el tumor.

EXERCISE 5-2

1. El loro ha mejorado un poco.
2. El perro no ha vomitado hoy. *Or* Hoy el perro no ha vomitado.
3. La yegua ha cojeado desde entonces.
4. Los gatitos han perdido peso.
5. El quiste ha crecido.
6. Los ácaros casi han desparecido.
7. He revisado los resultados.
8. La cerda ha parido.
9. El hinchazón ha diminuido.
10. Las vitaminas han ayudado mucho.

EXERCISE 5-3

Hace casi seis días que Happy está enfermo. Hace tres días que no come mucho y ha vomitado dos veces, pero ha bebido/tomado mucho agua. Hoy no ha comido y hace cinco horas que no orina. Creo que su condición ha empeorado.

EXERCISE 5-4

1. No les hemos dado vitaminas a los gatitos.
2. Usted no debe sobrealimentar a su animal.
3. Padece de la carencia de hierro.
4. Quiero darle una dieta balanceada.
5. ¿Podemos darle los obsequios?
6. Señor García, ¿le da usted la comida seca o la comida enlatada?
7. ¿Qué suplementos le ha dado usted?
8. Les he dado el maíz hasta este año.
9. ¿Qué le debemos darle de comer?
10. Hace dos días que tiene indigestión.

EXERCISE 5-5

1. Hace tres días que la vaca tiene aversión por el alimento. *Or* Hace tres días.
2. Sí, les doy vitaminas.
3. Le doy el heno y los suplementos.
4. Están a pasto.
5. Ha comido un GI Joe.
6. Consiste en la comida seca.
7. No le doy muchos. Le doy diez.
8. Sí, les doy suficiente sal. Tienen una salegar.

EXERCISE 6-1

1. parió
2. recibieron
3. descubrió
4. observó, ordeñó
5. diagnosticó, eliminaron, vacunaron
6. realizó
7. desinfecté, vendé
8. evaluamos, decidimos
9. presentó, mostró
10. bañó
11. sometió
12. pareció, picó
13. revisó
14. añadimos
15. subió

EXERCISE 6-2

1. el gato empieza, el gato empezó
2. los especialistas recomiendan, recomendaron

3. el potrillo duerme, durmió
4. el perro muerde, mordió
5. la paloma vuela, voló
6. las llamas siguen, siguieron
7. el maíz cuesta, costó
8. el laboratorio pide, pidió
9. los canarios mueren, murieron
10. el problema vuelve, volvió

EXERCISE 6-3

1. Le doy la melaza. Le di la melaza.
2. La secreción es abundante. La secreción fue abundante.
3. La situación está grave. La situación estuvo grave.
4. El ejercicio hace el problema peor. El ejercicio hizo el problema peor.
5. Tienen las vacunas regulares. Tuvieron las vacunas regulares.

EXERCISE 6-4

1. Examino el rebaño del señor Vivaldi todos los años. Voy a examinar el rebaño del señor Vivaldi mañana. Examiné el rebaño del señor Vivaldi ayer. Ya he examinado el rebaño del señor Vivaldi.
2. Las pruebas han mostrado la carencia de magnesio. Las pruebas muestran la carencia de magnesio. Las pruebas mostraron la carencia de magnesio. Las pruebas van a mostrar la carencia de magnesio.
3. Este medicamento expulsa los parásitos. Este medicamento expulsó los parásitos. Este medicamento va a expulsar los parásitos. Este medicamento ha expulsado los parásitos.
4. Ahora le damos una inyección. La semana pasada, le dimos una inyección. Después, vamos a darle una inyección. Le hemos dado una inyección.
5. Ahora come normalmente *or* come normalmente ahora. Comió normalmente hasta ayer. Hoy ha comido normalmente. Va a comer normalmente dentro de poco.

EXERCISE 6-5

1. Se tragó un alambre.
2. Se le infectó la herida.
3. Se cayó en un hoyo.
4. Se cortó con un clavo.
5. Se le rompió la costilla.
6. Se tomó el anticongelante.
7. Le atropelló una motocicleta.
8. Le picó una culebra/una serpiente.
9. Se le dañó el ala.
10. Mi nietito le dio aspirina.

EXERCISE 7-1

1. Sí, la tiene. No, no la tiene.
2. Sí, las toman. No, no las toman.
3. Sí, lo come. No, no lo come.
4. Sí, los receto. No, no los receto.
5. Sí, lo desinfecté. No, no lo desinfecté.
6. Sí, las pesé. No, no las pesé.
7. Sí, la toma. No, no la toma.
8. Sí, la tiene. No, no la tiene.
9. Sí, lo he notado. No, no lo he notado.
10. Sí, las recibieron. No, no las recibieron.

EXERCISE 7-2

1. espere
2. doble
3. tome
4. añada
5. describa
6. abra
7. proceda
8. lea
9. olvide
10. cambie
11. empiece
12. vuelva

EXERCISE 7-3

1. Dígame. No me diga.
2. Póngalos aquí. No los ponga aquí.
3. Tómela. No la tome.
4. Inyéctela. No la inyecte.
5. Descríbalos. No los describa.

EXERCISE 7-4

1. Give <u>the goat</u> a carrot.
2. Give <u>it</u> more salt.
3. Tell <u>me</u> the problem.
4. Write <u>him</u> a report.
5. Inject <u>it</u> with the vaccine.

EXERCISE 7-5

1. Dele una pastilla todos los días.
2. Dígale el problema.
3. Descríbame los signos.
4. Deme el termómetro, por favor.
5. Muéstreme la llaga.
6. No les dé sobras.
7. Ya no le recete los antibióticos.

EXERCISE 7-6

1. Es importante que usted los limpie regularmente.
2. No es necesario que Patches pase la noche en la clínica.
3. Recomiendo que usted consulte con un optamólogo veterinario.
4. La especialista/El especialista sugiere que tomemos rayos x.
5. Es important que usted desinfecte el ombligo.
6. No recomiendo que usted cambie su dieta.
7. Es importante que no rasgue la herida. [The *u* keeps the *g*, when followed by an *e*, from sounding like *j*.]
8. Sugiero que cubra used el área con ungüento.
9. Es important que Maddie no la lama.
10. Es necesario que Bubbles pierda peso.

Dictionary

alpiste, el—birdseed

already—*ya*

also—*también*

amarillento, amarillenta—yellowish

amarillo, amarilla—yellow

amino acid—*el aminoácido*

ampolla, la—blister

añadir—to add

análisis, el—analysis

analizar—to analyze

analysis—*el análisis*

analyze—*analizar*

anemia—*la anemia*

anemic—*anémico, anémica*

anémico, anémica—anemic

animal—*el animal*; small animals—*las pequeñas especies*; large animals—*las grandes especies*

ano, el—anus

año, el—year

anoche—last night

anormal—not normal, abnormal

anteayer—day before yesterday

antelope—*el antílope*

anteriormente—previously

antes—before

antibiotic—*el antibiótico*

antelope—*el antílope*

antifreeze—*el anticongelante*; It drank antifreeze.—*Se tragó el anticongelante.*

antílope, el—antelope

antimange medicine—*el antisárnico*

antisárnico, el—antimange medicine

antitetánico, el—tetanus shot

anus—*el ano*

apetito, el—appetite

aplicación, la—application

aplicar—to apply

apoyarse más—to favor; *Se apoya más en esta pata.*—It favors this paw.

appear—*parecer* (seem to, be similar to); *mostrar* (ue) (show signs of); *presentar* (show signs of). It appears it has a fever.—*Parece que tiene fiebre* or *Muestra fiebre* or *Presenta fiebre.*

appetite—*el apetito*

apple—*la manzana*

application—*la aplicación*

apply—*aplicar*

arañar—to scratch (with claws) to draw blood; *El gato le arañó al perro.*—The cat scratched the dog.

area—*el área, las áreas*

arena, la—kitty litter

arrhythmia—*la arritmia*

arrhythmic—*arrítmico, arrítmica*

arritmia, la—arrythmia

arrítmico, arrítmica—arrhythmic

arroyo, el—ditch; *Se cayó en el arroyo.*—It fell in a ditch.

arthritis—*la artritis*

artificial insemination—*la inseminación artificial*

artritis, la—arthritis

asa trompas, la—pig snare

ask (a question)—*preguntar*

ask for—*pedir* (i, i)

assail—*embestir* (i, i)

atactic—*atáxica, atáxico*

atáxica, atáxico—atactic

atención—attention, care; *con atención*—carefully, closely; *Observe la marcha con atención.*—Watch its gait closely.

atropellar—to run over; *Le atropelló un auto.*—A car ran over it.

autosuficiente—self-sufficient, independent

ave, el, las aves—bird, birds

ave de jaula, el, las aves de jaula—caged birds; pet birds

ave de rapiña, el, las aves de rapiña—bird of prey

avena, la—oats

aversión por el alimento, la—refusal to eat, aversion to food

avestruz, el—ostrich

avian—*aviar*

aviar—avian

avispa, la—wasp

ayer—yesterday

ayudar—to help

azul—blue

B

bad—*malo, mala*; a bad case—*un caso malo*; (condition) *mal*; My cow is bad off.—*La vaca está mal.*

bajar—to reduce, to lessen, to go down
(fever)

balanceado, balanceada—balanced

balanced—*balanceado, balanceada*;
equilibrado, equilibrada; a balanced
diet—*una dieta balanceada*

balar—to bleat

bald—*calvo, calva*

baldness—*la calvicie*

ballena, la—whale

ballico, el—ryegrass

bañar—to bathe, to dip

bandada, la—flock (of birds)

bandage—verb, *vendar*; noun, *la venda, el
vendaje*. Change the bandages once a
day—*Cambie la venda una vez al día.*

baño, el—bath; *el baño de inmersión*—
dipping bath

barbed wire—*el alambre*

bark—*ladrar*

barley—*la cebada*

barnyard—*el corral*

barrow—*el cerdo castrado*

batir—to beat (wings)

be—*ser* (for physical characteristics,
professions, or personality traits); *estar*
(for changeable conditions); both *ser*
and *estar* are irregular verbs

beak—*el pico*

bear—*el oso*

beat—*latir* (heart), *batir* (wings)

bebedero, el—water trough, water dish

beber—to drink

because (for the reason of)—*porque, debido
a*

becerrera, la—calf hutch

becerro, el, la becerra—calf

bee—*la abeja*

beef cattle—*el ganado de carne*

before—*antes, anteriormente*

begin—*comenzar* (ie), *empezar* (ie)

beginning—*el comienzo*

behavior—*el comportamiento*

believe—*creer*; I believe it has anemia.—
Creo que tiene anemia.

bend—*doblar*

benign—*benigno, benigna*; a benign
tumor—*un tumor benigno*

benigno, benigna—benign

best—*el mejor, la mejor*; what's best—*lo
mejor*

better—*mejor*; to get better—*mejorar*

bien—fine, well; ¿*Cómo está usted? Bien,
grácias.*—How are you? Fine, thank
you.

big—*grande*

biopsy—*la biopsia*; to take a biopsy—*sacar
una biopsia*

bird—*el pájaro, el ave (las aves)*; pet birds,
caged birds—*las aves de jaula*

bird of prey—*el ave de rapiña*

birdseed—*el alpiste*

birth—*el parto*; give birth—*parir* (animals
only). In humans, *dar a luz.*

bitch—*la perra*

bite—noun, *la mordida*; verb, *morder* (ue);
for snakes, *picar*

black—*negro, negra*

bladder—*la vesícula*; gallbladder—*la
vesícula biliar*; urinary bladder—*la
vesícula urinaria*

blanco, blanca—white

bleat—*balar*

bleed—*sangrar*

blind—*ciego, ciega*

blister—noun, *la ampolla*

bloated—*timpanizado, timpanizada*

blood—*la sangre*

blood poisoning—*la septicemia*

blood test—*el examen sanguíneo*

bloody—*sanguinolento, sanguinolenta*

blue—*azul*

boar—*el verraco*

boca, la—mouth

bola, la—lump

bola de pelo, la—fur ball

bonemeal—*la harina de huesos*

botana, la—treat (for pets)

botella, la—bottle

bottle—*la botella*

brain—*el cerébro, el encéfalo*

brand—*la marca*

branding—*el marcaje*

break—*romperse*; It broke its leg.—*Se le
rompió la pierna.*

breath—*la respiración*

breathe—*respirar*

breed—noun, *la raza*; verb, *criar, engendrar, procrear*

brewer's yeast—*la levadura de cerveza*

brown—*marrón; pardo, parda* (see also *café*)

brush—noun, *el cepillo;* verb, *cepillar*

buche, el—crop, craw

buck (male goat)—*el macho cabrío*

buey, el—ox

bull—*el toro*

burro, el—donkey

buy—*comprar*

C

caballeriza, la—stall

caballo, el—horse; *el caballo castrado*—gelding

cabeza, la—head

cable eléctrico, el—electrical wire

cabra, la—goat (female)

cabrito, el, la cabrita—kid (young goat)

cacatúa, la—cockatoo

cachexic—*caquéxico, caquéxica*

cachorro, el, la cachorra—puppy, cub

cactus—*el cacto, el cactus*; prickly pear cactus—*el nopal*

caer—to fall; *caerse*—to fall down

café—coffee-colored

calcio, el—calcium

calcium—*el calcio*; calcium deficiency—*la carencia de calcio*

calf—*el ternero, la ternera; el becerro, la becerra*

calf hutch—*la becerrera*

call—*llamar*; Call me if there are problems.—*Llámeme si hay problemas.*

calostro, el—colostrum

calvicie, la—baldness

calvo, calva—bald

camada, la—litter (of baby animals)

cambiar—to change

cambio, el—noun, change; *¿Notó un cambio?*—Did you notice a change?

camel—*el camello*

camello, el—camel

caminar—to walk

can, able to, may—*poder* (ue)

caña, la—shank

canary—*el canario*

cancer—*el cáncer*

canceroso, cancerosa—cancerous

cancerous—*canceroso, cancerosa*

canine—*canino, canina*

canino, canina—canine

canned food—*la comida enlatada*

cansar—to tire

capado, capada—castrated

capar—to castrate

caparazón, el—shell (turtle, tortoise)

caquéxico, caquéxica—cachexic

carcinoma—*el carcinoma*

care—noun, *el cuidado*

care for—verb, *cuidar de*

careful, be—*tener cuidado*; Be careful with the bandage.—*Tenga cuidado con la venda.*

carefully—*con cuidado*

carencia, la—deficiency; *carencia nutricional*—nutritional deficiency; *carencia de calcio*—calcium deficiency

carnero, el—ram, male sheep

carrot—*la zanahoria*

carry out (a task)—*cumplir, realizar*

cáscara, la—shell (egg)

casco, el—hoof; also, *la pezuña*

case (medical)—*el caso*; It's a difficult case.—*Es un caso difícil.*

caseta, la—stall

caso, el—case (medical)

castrado, castrada—castrated

castrar—to castrate

castrate—*capar, castrar*

castrated—*capado, capada; castrado, castrada*

cattle—noun, *el ganado*; adjective, *ganadero, ganadera*

causa, la—noun, cause

causar—to cause

cause—noun, *la causa*; verb, *causar*

cebada, la—barley

cebra, la—zebra

celo, el—rut, in season. *Está en celo.*—It's in season.

cepillar—to brush

cepillo, el—noun, brush

cerda de remplazo, la—gilt

cerdo, el, la cerda—pig; *el cerdo castrado*—barrow; *cerdo en crecimiento, el*—growing swine; *cerdo en finalización*—finishing swine

cereal—*el cereal*

cerebral—*cerebral*

cerebro, el—brain

change—verb, *cambiar*; noun, *el cambio*

check, check over—*revisar* (test results)

chew—*masticar*; chew through (a wire)—*morder* (ue)

chichón, el—lump

chick—*el pollito, la pollita*; (pet birds) *el polluelo, la polluela*

chicken—noun, *el gallo, la gallina*; adjective, *aviar*

chicken cholera—*el cólera aviar*

chine—*el lomo*

chivo, el; la chiva—kid (young goat); kid (human)—*el niño, la niña; el muchacho, la muchacha*

cholera—*el cólera*

chorro, el—stream (of urine)

chronic—*crónico, crónica*

cianótico, cianótica—cyanotic

ciego, ciega—blind

ciencia, la—science, knowledge

ciervo, el; la cierva—deer

cinco—five

circle—*el círculo*; to walk in circles—*marchar en círculos*

círculo, el—circle

cirugía, la—surgery

claro, clara—clear

claw—noun, *la garra*; verb, *arañar*

clean—adjective, *limpio, limpia*; verb, *limpiar*

clear—*claro, clara*

client—*el cliente, la clienta*

clinic—*la clínica*

clínica, la—clinic

clinical—*clínico, clínica*

clinical history—*el historial clínico*

clínico, clínica—clinical

clip—noun, *el corte*; nail clip—*el corte de uñas*; verb, *cortar*

clip the needle teeth—*descolmillar*

closely (cautiously)*con atención*; Read the label closely.—*Lea la etiqueta con atención.*

cloudy—*turbio, turbia*

clover—*el trébol*

cobaya, la—guinea pig

cochinillo, el, la cochinilla—piglet

cockatoo—*la cacatúa*

cocodrilo, el—crocodile

cod liver oil—*el aceite de hígado de bacalao*

coffee-colored—*café*

cojear—to limp

cojo, coja—lame; *Está cojo.*—It's lame.

cola, la—tail

colapsado, colapsada—collapsed

cólera, el—cholera; *el cólera aviar*—avian cholera

colic—*el cólico*

cólico, el—colic

collapsed—*colapsado, colapsada*

colon—*el colon*

color—*el color*

colostrum—*el calostro*

colt—*el potro, la potranca*

comb—(cockscomb) *la cresta*; (for grooming) *el peine*

come back—*volver (ue), regresar*; Come back tomorrow.—*Vuelva usted mañana.*

comedero, el—food trough, food dish

comenzar (ie)—to begin

comer—to eat

comida, la—food

comida enlatada, la—canned food

comida húmeda, la—wet food

comida seca, la—dry food

comienzo, el—beginning

comportamiento, el—behavior

comprar—to buy

comprender—to understand

concentrado, concentrada—concentrated

concentrate—noun, *el concentrado*

concentrated—*concentrado, concentrada*

condición, la—condition

condition—*la condición*

conducto glactóforo, el—milk duct

conejillo de Indias, el—guinea pig

conejo, el, la coneja—rabbit
congested—*congestionado, congestionada*
congestionado, congestionada—congested
conjunctivitis—*la conjunctivitis*
consist of—*consistir en*
consistir en—consist of
costilla, la—rib
continue—*seguir* (i, i); Continue the
　treatment.—*Siga el tratamiento.*
constipación, la—constipation
consult—*consultar*
consulta, la—consultation; *horas de
　consulta*—office hours
consultar—to consult
contagious—*contagioso, contagiosa*
control—noun, *el control*; verb, *controlar*
control, el—control, barrier, checkpoint
controlar—to control
convulsiones, las—convulsions; seizures
convulsions—*las convulsiones*
coordinación, la—coordination; *la
　incoordinación*—lack of coordination
coordination—*la coordinación*; lack of
　coordination—*la incoordinación*
corazón, el—heart
cordero, el, la cordera—lamb
corn—*el maíz*
coronilla, la—poll
corral—*el corral*
correr—to run (not walk)
cortar—to cut, to clip
cortarse—to cut oneself; *Se cortó con un
　alambre.*—It cut itself on barbed wire.
corte, el—the cut, the cutting; the clip, the
　clipping
corvejón, el—hock; also, *el tarso*
cosecha, la—crop (agricultural product)
cost—noun, *el costo, el precio*; verb, *costar*
　(ue); It doesn't cost much.—*No cuesta
　mucho.*
costar (ue)—to cost
cotton, cottonseed—*el algodón*
cottonseed cake—*la torta de algodón*
cough—noun, *la tos*; verb, *toser*; Does it
　cough?—*¿Tiene tos?*; to cough up
　(blood)—*toser con (sangre)*; to cough up
　a fur ball—*vomitar la bola de pelo*

cover—verb, *cubrir*; regular except for the
　present perfect: *he cubierto*
cow—*la vaca*
craw—*el buche*
crecer—to grow
creer—to believe, to think
crest—*la cresta*
cresta, la—comb (cockscomb); crest
cría, la—offspring
criar—to breed, to raise
crocodile—*el cocodrilo*
crónico, crónica—chronic
crop—noun, (of a bird) *el buche*;
　(agricultural product) *la cosecha*; verb,
　cortar, recortar, amputar, desmochar (the
　tail of a horse)
cruz, la—withers
cruzado, el, la cruzada—mutt
cuando, ¿Cuándo?—when
¿Cuánto?—how many? how much?
cuartilla, la—pastern
cuatro—four
cub—*el cachorro, la cachorra*
cubrir—to cover; regular except for the
　present perfect: *he cubierto*
cuello, el—neck
cuerno, el—horn
cuerpo extraño, el—foreign body
cuidado, el—care, caution; *con cuidado*—
　carefully; *tener cuidado*—to be careful
cuidar de—to care for
culebra, la—snake
cumplir—to reach, to achieve, to carry out
curar—to cure
cure—verb, *curar, remediar*; noun, *el
　remedio*
cut—*cortar, mochar*; to cut off—*recortar,
　amputar, desmochar* (the tail of a horse)
cuy, el—guinea pig
cyanotic—*cianótico, cianótica*
cyst—*el quiste*

D_____

daily—adjective, *diario, diaria*; daily
　food—*la comida diaria*; adverb,
　diariamente; Brush the puppy daily.—
　Cepille al perrito diariamente.

dairy—*la lechería*

dairy cattle—*el ganado de leche*; dairy cows—*las vacas lecheras*

damage—verb, *dañar, lastimar*

dañar—to damage

dar (an irregular verb)—to give

dar de comer (*dar* is an irregular verb)—to feed

dark—*oscuro, oscura*

day—*el día*

day after tomorrow—*pasado mañana*

day before yesterday—*anteayer*

deaf—*sordo, sorda*

deafness—*la sordera*

deber—ought to, should; *Usted debe suplementar la dieta de la vaca.*—You should supplement the cow's diet.

debido a—due to, because of

decir (an irregular verb)—to tell, to say; *Dígame el problema.*—Tell me the problem.

dedo, el—toe

deer—*el venado, el ciervo*

defecar—to defecate

defecate—*defecar*

defects—*los defectos*

deficiency—*la carencia*; calcium deficiency—*la carencia de calcio*

dehorn—*descornar* (ue)

dehydration—*la deshidratación*

demasiado, demasiada—too, too much

dense—*espeso, espesa*

depend—*depender*; to depend on—*depender de*

depender—to depend; *depender de*—to depend on

dermatitis—*la dermatitis*

derramar—to spill, to flow (implies more quantity than just a discharge or drainage)

decide—*decidir*

decidir—to decide

decision—*la decisión*

desaparecer—to disappear

descolar—to dock (the tail of sheep)

descolmillar—to clip the needle teeth

descornar (ue)—to dishorn, to dehorn, to disbud

describir—to describe

descubrir—to discover; regular except in present perfect: *he descubierto*

deshidratación, la—dehydration

desinfectar—to disinfect

desmochar—to crop (the tail of a horse)

desnutrición, la—malnutrition

despacio—slow, slowly

desparasitar—to worm, to rid of parasites

después—after, later

destetar—to wean

destete, el—weaning

dewlap—*la papada*

día, el—day

diagnose—*diagnosticar*

diagnosis—*el diagnóstico*

diagnosticar—to diagnose

diagnóstico, el—diagnosis

diariamente—(adv.) daily, every day

diario, diaria—daily

diarrea, la—diarrhea

diarrhea—*la diarrea*

die—*morir* (ue, u); also irregular in the present perfect: The fish has died.—*El pez ha muerto.*

diet—*la dieta, el régimen*

dieta, la—diet

diez—ten

difficult—*difícil; dificultoso, dificultosa*

difficulty—*la dificultad*; to have difficulty breathing—*tener dificultad para respirar*

difícil—hard (difficult)

dificultad, la—difficulty

dificultoso, dificultosa—difficult

difteria, la—dyphtheria

digerir (ie, i)—to digest

digest—*digerir* (ie, i)

digestion—*la digestión*

digestive—*digestivo, digestiva*

diminish—*disminuir*

dip—verb, *bañar*; noun, *el baño*

dipping bath—*el baño de inmersión*

disappear—*desaparecer*

disbud—*descornar* (ue)

discharge—noun, (without pus) *la secreción, el escurrimiento*; It has a discharge from the eyes.—*Tiene secreción ocular*; (with pus) *la supuración*; verb, (with pus) *supurar*; There is a discharge from the vagina.—*Le supura la vagina.*; *escurrir*—to drain; *derramar*—to spill, to flow (implies more quantity than a secretion or drainage)

discover—*descubrir*; regular except for the present perfect: *he descubierto*

disentería, la—dysentery

disinfect—*desinfectar*

dislocation—*la dislocación*

disminuir—to diminish, to shrink

disnea, la—dyspnea

disolución, la—solution (dissolved in liquid)

disparar—to shoot; *Le disparó un cazador.*—A hunter shot it.

distemper—*el moquillo, el distémper*

distended—*distendido, distendida*

distensión, la—distension

ditch—*el arroyo*; It fell in a ditch.—*Se cayó en el arroyo.*

do (carry out an action)—*hacer* (an irregular verb); not used to make a question: Do you give it vitamins?—*¿Le da vitaminas?*

doblar—to bend (something); to turn (the corner); to fold

doce—twelve

docile—*manso, mansa*

dock—*descolar*

dog—*el perro, la perra*

dolor, el—pain; *con dolor*—painfully

domingo, el—Sunday

donde, ¿Dónde?—where

donkey—*el burro, la burra*

dormir (ue, u)—to sleep

dos—two

dose—noun, *la dósis*; verb, *dosificar*

dosificar—to dose

dósis, la—dose

dos veces—twice

down (go down)—*bajar*; The fever has gone down.—*Ha bajado la fiebre.*

down (lying down)—*tumbado, tumbada*

drain—*escurrir*

drainage—(without pus) *el escurrimiento, la secreción*; (with pus) *la supuración*; (more quantity) *el derrame*

dress (a wound)—*vendar*

drink—*beber, tomar*

drops—*las gotas*; Put these drops in its eye.—*Ponga estas gotas en el ojo.*

dry—*seco, seca*

dry food—*la comida seca, la comida desecada*

due to—*debido a, porque*

dueño, el, dueña, la—owner

duro, dura—hard (not soft)

dying—*moribundo, moribunda*

dyphtheria—*la difteria*

dysentery—*la disentería*

E

ear—*la oreja* (external part); *el oído* (internal part)

ear marking, notching—*el mosqueo*

easily—*fácilmente*

easy—*fácil*

eat—*comer*

edad, la—age

efecto, el—effect

effect—*el efecto*

egg—*el huevo*

eggshell—*la cáscara*

eight—*ocho*

ejercicio, el—exercise

electrical wire—*el cable eléctrico*

elefante, el—elephant

elephant—*el elefante*

elevado, elevada—elevated

elevated—*elevado, elevada*

eliminar—to eliminate

eliminate—*eliminar*

embestir—to assail

empeorar—to worsen

empezar (ie)—to begin

empty—*vacío, vacía*

encéfalo, el—brain

encephalus—*el encéfalo*

encías, las—gums

encojido, encojida—hunched (posture)

endemic—*endémico, endémica*
energetic—*activo, activa*
energía, la—energy
energy—*la energía*
enfermedad, la—sickness, illness; *la enfermedad hepática*—liver disease; *la enfermedad hemolítica*—hemolytic disease*
enfermero, el, la enfermera—nurse
enfermo, enferma—sick, ill
engendrar—to breed
engordar—to fatten
enjuage de los pezones, el—teat dipping
enlatado, enlatada—canned; *la comida enlatada*—canned food
enrojecido, enrojecida—reddened
ensilaje, el—silage
enterovirus—*el enterovirus*
entumecido, entumecida—swollen; also *hinchado, hinchada*
enzima, la—enzyme
enzyme—*la enzima*
epidemia, la—epidemic
epidemic—*la epidemia*
equine—*equino, equina*
equino, equina—equine
erisipela, la—erysipelas
erysipelas—*la erisipela*
escaso, escasa—scant, not much, scarce
escofinar—to rasp
escribir—to write; regular except in the present perfect: *He escrito*
escroto, el—scrotum
escuchar—to listen
escurrimiento, el—drainage, discharge without pus
esófago, el—esophagus
esophagus—*el esófago*
especialista, el, la especialista—specialist
especie, la—species, type
esperar—to wait, to wait for; *Por favor, espere aquí.*—Please wait here.
espeso, espesa—thick, dense, clotted
espina, la—thorn
esporádico, esporádica—sporadic
esposo, el, la esposa—husband, wife
espuma, la—foam

estable—stable (not changing)
establo, el—stable (barn)
estabulado, estabulada—stabled, kept in a stable
esta mañana—this morning
esta noche—tonight
esta tarde—this afternoon, this evening
estar (an irregular verb)—to be (used for changeable conditions); *La vaca está enferma.*—The cow is sick.
este, esta—this; this morning—*esta mañana*
esteemed—*estimado, estimada*
estéril—sterile, not fertile
estimado, estimada—esteemed
estómago, el—stomach
evaluar—to evaluate; to examine
evaluate—*evaluar*
every day—*todos los días; diariamente*
ewe—*la oveja*
exam, examination—*el examen*
examen, el—exam
examen sanguíneo, el—blood test
examinar—to examine
examination—*el examen, la evaluación*
examine—*examinar, evaluar, revisar*
excremento, el—excrement, stool
exercise—*el ejercicio*
expel (parasites)—*expulsar*
expulsar—to expel (parasites)
extend—*extender* (ie); Extend its wing please.—*Por favor, extienda el ala.*
extender (ie)—to extend, to stretch out
external—*externo, externa*
externo, externa—external
extraño, extraña—strange, odd; *el cuerpo extraño*—foreign body
eye—*el ojo*

F_____
fácil—easy
fácilmente—easily
failure—*la falla*; kidney failure—*la falla renal*
fall—verb, *caer*; to fall down—*caerse*; noun, *la caída*
falla, la—failure; *la falla renal*—kidney failure

falta, la—noun, lack; lack of exercise—*la falta de ejercicio*

faltar—verb, to lack; *Le falta la proteína.*— It lacks protein.

faringe, la—mouth

farm—*la granja, la finca*; poultry farm—*la granja avícola*

farrow—*parir*; farrowing—*el parto*

fat—noun, *la grasa*; milkfat—*la grasa láctea*; adjective, *gordo, gorda*

fatten—*engordar*

fatty tumor—*el tumor grasoso*

favor (one foot)—*apoyarse más (en una pata)*

feather—*la pluma*; plumage—*el plumaje*

feces—*las heces*

fecundo, fecunda—fertile

feed—noun, *la comida, el alimento, el pienso*; verb, *dar de comer, alimentar*; overfeed—*sobrealimentar*

feed trough, feed bowl—*el comedero*

feline—*felino, felina*

feline leukemia—*la leucemia felina*

felino, felina—feline

female—*la hembra*

fertile—*fértil, fecundo, fecunda*

fetid—*fétido, fétida*

fetlock—*el menudillo*

fever—*la fiebre*

few—*poco, poca*

fewer—*menos*

fiebre, la—fever

fiebre aftosa, la—hoof and mouth disease

fiebre vitularia, la—milk fever

fifteen—*quince*

fight—*pelear*

filly—*la potranca*

finca, la—farm

fine—*bien*; How are you? Fine, thanks.— *¿Cómo está usted? Bien, gracias.*

finish (a task)—*terminar*

finishing swine—*el cerdo en finalización*

fish—noun, *el pez*; (on a plate) *el pescado*; verb, *pescar*

físico, física—physical

five—*cinco*

flaco, flaca—thin, skinny

flanco, el—flank

flank—*el flanco*

flea—*la pulga*

flema, la—phlegm

flock—(of sheep) *el rebaño*; (of chickens) *la parvada, la gallinería*; (of birds) *la bandada*

fly—noun, *la mosca*; horn fly—*la mosca del cuerno*; verb, *volar* (ue)

foal—noun, *el potrillo, la potranquita*; verb, *parir*

foam—*la espuma*

fodder—*el forraje*

following, following manner—*siguiente; la siguiente manera*

food—*el alimento*

food bowl, food trough—*el comedero*

foot—*el pie, la pata* (paw)

forage—*el forraje*

foreign body—*el cuerpo extraño*

forget—*olvidarse*; Don't forget to call.—*No se olvide de llamar.*

forraje, el—fodder, forage

foul-smelling—*fétido, fétida*

four—*cuatro*

fox—*el zorro*

fractura, la—fracture

fracture—noun, *la fractura*; verb, *romperse, fracturarse*; It fractured a leg.—*Se le rompió la pierna; Se le fracturó la pierna.*

frecuente—frequent; opposite: *infrequente*

frecuentemente—frequently

frequent—*frecuente*; opposite: *infrequente*

frequently—*frecuentemente*

fresco, fresca—fresh

fresh—*fresco, fresca*; fresh fruit—*la fruta fresca*

Friday—*el viernes*

frog—*la rana*

fungus—*los hongos*

fur—*el pelo*; furs (for clothing)—*las pieles*

fur ball—*la bola de pelo*

G

gain—*ganar*; to gain weight—*ganar peso*; *engordar*

gait—*la marcha*

gallbladder—*la vesícula biliar*
galletitas, las—treats (for pets)
gallina, la—hen
gallinería, la, la parvada—flock of chickens
gallo, el—rooster
ganadero, ganadera—adjective, cattle; *la industria ganadera*—the cattle industry
ganado, el—noun, cattle
ganar—to gain
gangrena, la—gangrene
gangrene—*la gangrena*
garañón, el—stallion
garguero, el—gullet
garra, la—claw, talon
garrapata, la—tick; *las garrapatas ixodes*—ixodid ticks
gato, el, la gata—cat
gelding—*el caballo castrado*
gender—*el género*; sex—*el sexo*
género, el—gender; *el sexo*—sex
gestación, la—gestation, pregnancy
gestante—pregnant
gestation—*la gestación*
get better—*mejorar*
get up, stand up—*levantarse*
gilt—*la cerda de remplazo*
giraffe—*la jirafa*
give—*dar* (an irregular verb); to give birth—*parir*
gizzard—*la molleja*
gland—*la glándula*; adrenal gland—*la glándula adrenal*
glándula, la—gland
glándula adrenal, la—adrenal gland
glandular—*glandular*
go—*ir* (an irregular verb); going to (do something)—*ir a* + infinitive; I'm going to examine the eye.—*Voy a examinar el ojo.*
go over (test results or case history)—*revisar*
go up, rise—*subir*
goat—*la cabra* (female); *el macho cabrío* or *el cabra macho* (male)
gordo, gorda—adjective, fat
gotas, las—drops
gradually—*gradualmente*

gradualmente—gradually
grande—big
granja, la—farm; *la granja avícola*—poultry farm
grasa, la—noun, fat; *la grasa láctea*—milkfat
grass—*la hierba, el pasto, la yerba*
grave—serious, grave; *un caso grave*—a serious case; close to death; *La vaca está grave.*—The cow is close to death.
graze—*pacer, pastar*
grazing—*el pastoreo*
grazing cattle—*el ganado en pastoreo*
grazing land—*el pasto*
green—*verde*
grit (for birds)—*el grit*
grow—*crecer*
growing swine—*el cerdo en crecimiento*
grupa, la—rump
guinea pig—*el conejillo de Indias, el cuy; la cobaya*; guinea pig (in Mexico)—*el cuyo*
gullet—*el garguero*
gums—*las encías*
gusano, el—worm; also, *la lombriz*

H

habit—*el hábito, la costumbre*
hábito, el—habit; also *la costumbre*
hablar—to speak; *Por favor, hable más despacio.*—Speak more slowly, please.
hacer (an irregular verb)—to do, to make
happen—*pasar, ocurrir, suceder;* What happened?—*¿Qué pasó?*
hard—(not soft) *duro, dura*; (difficult) *difícil*
hardware disease—*la reticuloperitonitis traumática*
harina, la—meal; *la harina de huesos*—bonemeal
hasta—until
have—*tener* (an irregular verb); have to (do something)—*tener que*; I have to finish this report.—*Tengo que terminar este informe.*
hay—there is, there are
hay—*el heno*
head—*la cabeza*

heart—*el corazón*
heartbeat—*el latido del corazón*
heart murmur—*el murmullo cardíaco*
heart rate—*el ritmo cardíaco*
heces, las—feces
heel—*el talón*
heifer—*la vaquilla*
help—(to assist) *ayudar*; (to make better)
  mejorar
hematuria, la—hematuria
hembra, la—female
hemofilia, la—hemophilia
hemolytic disease—*la enfermedad
  hemolítica*
hemorragia, la—hemorrhage
hemorrhage—noun, *la hemorragia*; verb,
  sangrar
hen—*la gallina*
heno, el—hay
herd (of horses)—*la manada*; (of pigs)—*la
  piara*
herida, la—injury, wound
hernia—*la hernia*
herradura, la—horseshoe
herraje, el—horseshoeing
hide—*la piel*
hierba, la—grass
hierba callera, la—sedum
hierro, el—iron; *la inyección de hierro*—iron
  shot
hígado, el—liver
hinchado, hinchada—swollen
hinchazón, el—swelling
hippopotamus—*el hipopótamo*
historial clínico, el—clinical history
history, clinical—*el historial clínico*
hocico, el—muzzle
hock—*el corvejón, el tarso*
hold still—*sostener* (small animals),
  conjugated like *tener*; *sujetar* (large
  animals)
hombro, el—shoulder
hongos, los—fungus
hoof—*la pezuña, el casco*
hoof and mouth disease—*la fiebre aftosa*
hora, la—hour
hormona, la—hormone

hormonal—*hormonal*
hormone—*la hormona*
horn—*el cuerno*
horse—*el caballo*
horseshoe—*la herradura*
horseshoeing—*el herraje*
hour—*la hora*
How long? (time)—*¿Cuánto tiempo?*
How many?—*¿Cuánto?*
hoy—today
huevo, el—egg
hump—*la joroba*
hunched—*encojido, encojida*
hundido, hundida—sunken
husband—*el esposo, el marido*

I

ill—*enfermo, enferma*
illness—*la enfermedad*
immune system—*el sistema inmune*
immunity—*la inmunidad*
impactado, impactada—impacted
impacted—*impactado, impactada*
important—*importante*
improve—*mejorar*
incontinence—*la incontinencia*
incontinencia, la—incontinence
incoordinación, la—lack of coordination
indicar—to indicate
indicate—*indicar*
indigestion—*la indigestión*
infección, la—infection
infect—*infectar*
infectar—to infect
infected—*infectado, infectada*
infection—*la infección*
infectious—*infeccioso, infecciosa*
infertile—*infértil, infecundo, infecunda,
  estéril*; opposite: *fértil, fecundo, fecunda*
infestation—*la infestación*
inflamado, inflamada—inflamed
inflamed—*inflamado, inflamada*
informe, el—noun, (written) report
infrecuente—infrequent
infrequent—*infrecuente*
inject—*inyectar*
injection—*la inyección*

injured—*lastimado, lastimada; herido, herida*

injury—*la herida*

inmunidad, la—immunity

inocular—to inoculate; *inocular contra*—to inoculate against

inoculate—*inocular*; to inoculate against—*inocular contra*

insect—*el insecto, el bicho*

inseminación, la—insemination; *la inseminación artificial*—artificial insemination

inseminar—to inseminate

inseminate—*inseminar*

insemination—*la inseminación*; artificial insemination—*la inseminación artificial*

insufficiency—*la insuficiencia*; heart insufficiency—*la insuficiencia cardíaca*

inteligente—intelligent

intelligent—*inteligente*

internal—*interno, interna*

interno, interna—internal

intestinal—*intestinal*

intestine—*el intestino*

intestino, el—intestine

introducir—to introduce, to squirt

inyección, la—injection

inyectar—to inject

iodine—*el yodo*

ir (an irregular verb)—to go; *ir a + infinitive*—going to (do something)

iron—*el hierro*; iron shot—*la inyección de hierro*

irregular—*irregular*; (heartbeat) *agitado, agitada*

isolate—*aislar, separar*

ixodicida, la—ixodicide

ixodicide—*la ixodicida*

ixodid ticks—*las garrapatas ixodes*

J

jadear—to pant

jaule, la—cage

jauría, la—pack (of dogs)

jinete, el, la jinete—rider (of horses)

jirafa, la—giraffe

joroba, la—hump

jueves, el—Thursday

jugular vein—*la vena yugular*

just, to have just (done something)—*acabar de*; Dr. García has just arrived.—*El doctor García acaba de llegar.*

K

keep—(doing something) *seguir (i, i)*; Keep giving it vitamins.—*Siga dándole vitaminas.*; (apart) *mantener*, conjugated like *tener*; Keep it apart from the others.—*Manténgalo separado de los demás.*

kennel—*la perrera*

keratitis—*la queratitis*

kid—(animal) *el cabrito, la cabrita; el chivo, la chiva*; (human) *el niño, la niña* (small children); *el muchacho, la muchacha* (adolescents)

kidney—noun, *el riñón*; adjective, *renal*

kitten—*el gatito, la gatita*

kitty litter—*la arena*

knee—*la rodilla*

L

laboratory—*el laboratorio*

lácteo, láctea—adjective, milk

lack—noun, *la falta (de energía); la carencia (de la vitamina C)*; verb, *faltar*; It lacks protein.—*Le falta la proteína.*

ladrar—to bark

lamb—*el cordero, la cordera*

lamer—to lick

laminitis—*la laminitis*

lana, la—wool

large animals—*las grandes especies*

lastimado, lastimada—injured

lastimar—to injure

last month—*el mes pasado*

last night—*anoche*

last week—*la semana pasada*

lately—*últimamente, recientemente*

latido del corazón, el—heartbeat

latir—to beat (heart)

lavar—to wash

lay eggs—*poner huevos*

leche, la—milk

lechera, la—milk-producing animal; *la vaca lechera*—milk cow; *la cabra lechera*—milk goat

lechería, la—dairy farm

lechón, el, la lechona—piglet, suckling pig

lechoso, lechosa—milky

lechuza, la—owl; also *el buho*

leer—to read

leftovers—*las sobras (de comida);* Don't give it leftovers.—*No le dé las sobras de comida.*

leg—*la pierna*

lentamente—slowly

león, el—lion

lesion—*la lesión*

less—*menos*

lessen—*bajar*

letárgico, letárgica—lethargic

letargo, el—lethargy

lethargic—*letárgico, letárgica; inactivo, inactiva*

lethargy—*el letargo; la falta de energía*

leucemia, la—leukemia

leukemia—*la leucemia;* feline leukemia—*la leucemia felina*

levadura de cerveza, la—brewer's yeast

levantarse—to get up, to stand up

lice—*los piojos*

lick—*lamer*

limp—adjective, *cojo, coja;* verb, *cojear*

limpiar—to clean

limpio, limpia—adjective, clean

lion—*el león*

listen—*escuchar*

litter—*la camada* (baby animals); kitty litter—*la arena*

live—verb, *vivir*

liver—*el hígado*

liver disease—*la enfermedad hepática*

llaga, la—sore, ulcer

llama—*la llama*

llamar—to call; Call me if it's worse.—*Llámeme si está peor.*

llano, el—plain, prairie

lloroso, llorosa—watery, teary

loin—*el lomo*

lombriz, la—worm, especially tapeworm

lo mejor—what's best

lomo, el—loin, chine

loro, el—parrot

lose—*perder* (ie); to lose weight—*perder peso*

loss—*la pérdida*

lots of, a lot—*mucho, mucha*

low—*bajo, baja;* opposite: *elevado, alto*

lower—verb, *bajar*

lump—*la bola, el chichón*

lunes, el—Monday

lung—*el pulmón*

lying down—*tumbado, tumbada*

M

macho—male; *hembra*—female

macho cabrío, el—male goat, buck

magnesio, el—magnesium

magnesium—*el magnesio;* magnesium deficiency—*la carencia de magnesio*

maíz, el—corn

mal—bad, badly, poorly; *La vaca está mal.*—The cow is doing poorly.

mal, el—illness, malady

malady—*el mal, la enfermedad*

male—*macho;* female—*hembra*

malignant—*maligno, maligna*

malnutrition—*la desnutrición*

mamífero, mamífera,—adjective, mammalian

mamífero, el—noun, mammal

mammal—noun, *el mamífero*

mammalian—adjective, *mamífero, mamífera*

manada, la—herd (of horses)

mañana, la—morning, tomorrow; *mañana por la noche*—tomorrow night; *mañana por la tarde*—tomorrow afternoon

manchado, manchada (de sangre)—stained, tinged, spotted (with blood)

mange—*la sarna;* antimange medicine—*el antisárnico*

manso, mansa—tame, docile

mantener (an irregular verb)—keep; *mantener separado(a)*—keep apart

manzana, la—apple

many—*mucho, mucha*
marca, la—brand
marcaje, el—the branding
marcha, la—gait
marchar—to walk; *marchar en círculos*—to walk in circles
mare—*la yegua*
marrón—brown; also *pardo, parda*
martes, el—Tuesday
más—more
más o menos—more or less
mascota, la—pet
mass—*la masa*; tissue mass—*la masa de tejido*
masticar—to chew
mastitis—*la mastitis*
maullar—to meow
medicamento, el—medicine (prescription)
medicine—(a prescription) *el medicamento*; (the science) *la medicina*
mejor—better, improved
mejorar—to get better, to improve
melaza, la—molasses
menudillo, el—fetlock
meow—verb, *maullar*; (sound) *miau*
mes, el—month
miércoles, el—Wednesday
mijo, el—millet
milk—adjective, *lácteo, láctea*; noun, *la leche*; verb, *ordeñar*; milk production—*la producción láctea*
milk cow—*la vaca lechera*
milk duct—*el conducto glactóforo*
milkfat—*la grasa láctea*
milk fever—*la fiebre vitularia; la fiebre de la leche*
milking shed—*el local de ordeño, la sala de ordeño*
milky—*lechoso, lechosa*
millet—*el mijo, el millo*
millo, el—millet
minerals—*los minerales*
minute—*el minuto*
minuto, el—minute
miscarriage—*el aborto*
mite—*el ácaro*
moco, el—mucus

modern—*moderno, moderna*
moderno, moderna—modern
molasses—*la melaza*
molleja, la—gizzard
moment—*el momento*; A moment, please.—*Un momento, por favor.*
momento, el—moment
Monday—*el lunes*
monkey—*el mono*
mono, el—monkey
monta, la—mounting; copulation
month—*el mes*; Come back in a month.—*Vuelva en un mes.*
moo—*mugir*
moquillo, el—distemper
morbid—*morboso, morbosa*
morboso, morbosa—morbid, badly ill
morder (ue)—to bite
more—*más*
mordida, la—bite
moribundo, moribunda—dying
morir (ue, u)—to die
mortinato, el—stillbirth
mosca, la—fly; *la mosca del cuerno*—horn fly
mosqueo, el—ear marking, notching
mostrar (ue)—to show, to appear, to show signs of
mounting (copulation)—*la monta*
mouth—*la boca, la faringe*
move—*mover (ue)*
mover (ue)—to move
muchacho, el, la muchacha—kid (human, adolescent)
mucho, mucha—many, a lot
mucosas, las—mucous membranes
mucosidad, la, el moco—mucus
mucous membranes—*las mucosas*
mucus—*el moco, la mucosidad*
muestra, la—sample
mugir—to moo
mule—*la mula*
murmur—*el murmullo*; heart murmur—*el murmullo cardíaco*
muscle—*el músculo*
músculo, el—muscle
mutt—*el cruzado, la cruzada*

muy—very
muzzle—*el hocico*

N

nail—(toe nail) *la uña*; (construction) *el clavo*
nail clip—*el corte de uñas*
nariz, la—nose
navel—*el ombligo*
necesario, necesaria—necessary
necesitar—to need
necessary—*necesario, necesaria*
neck—*el cuello*
need—verb, *necesitar*
negro, negra—black
neigh—*relinchar*
nerve—*el nervio*
nervio, el—nerve
nervous system—*el sistema nervioso*
neumonía, la—pneumonia (in animals; in humans, *la pulmonía*)
new—*nuevo, nueva*
newborn—*recién nacido, recién nacida*
next—*próximo, próxima*; next month—*el próximo mes*; next week—*la próxima semana*
nice—*simpático, simpática* (for humans only, not for objects)
nine—*nueve*
niños, los—children
noise—*el sonido, el ruido*
nopal, el—prickly pear cactus
normal—*normal*
normally—*normalmente*
normalmente—normally
nose—*la nariz*
nostril—*el ollar*
not—*no*; It is not leukemia.—*No es leucemia.*
notar—to notice
notice—*notar*
nourish—*alimentar, dar de comer*
novillo, el—steer
now—*ahora*
nueve—nine
nuevo, nueva—new
number—*el número*

número, el—number
nurse—*el enfermero, la enfermera*
nutrición, la—nutrition
nutrido, nutrida—nurtured, raised on
nutrition—*la nutrición, la alimentación*
nutritional—*nutricional, alimentario, alimentaria*
nutritional deficiency—*la carencia nutricional, la carencia alimentaria*

O

oats—*la avena*
obese—*obeso, obesa*
obeso, obesa—obese
obsequios, los—treats (for pets)
observar—to observe, to watch
observe—*observar*
ocho—eight
occur—*ocurrir, pasar*
ocurrir—to occur, to happen
odor—*el olor*; a bad odor—*un olor fétido*
office hours—*las horas de consulta*
offspring—*la cría*
oftalmólogo, el, la oftalmóloga—ophthalmologist
oído, el—ear (internal part)
oilcake—*la torta oleaginosa*
ointment—*el ungüento*
ojo, el—eye
oler (ue)—to smell, to have an odor; *La respiración huele mal.*—Its breath smells bad.
ollar, el—nostril
olor, el—odor; *un olor fétido*—a bad odor
olvidarse—to forget
ombligo, el—navel
once—*una vez*; once a day—*una vez al día*
one—*uno; un, una*
open—adjective, *abierto, abierta*; verb, *abrir*; regular except in the present perfect: *He abierto la botella.*—I have opened the bottle.
ophthalmologist—*el oftalmólogo, la oftalmóloga*
ordeñar—to milk
oreja, la—ear (external part)
orina, la—urine

orinar—to urinate

oscuro, oscura—dark

oso, el—bear

ostrich—*el avestruz*

ought to—*deber*

ovario, el—ovary

ovary—*el ovario*

oveja, la—ewe

overfeed—*sobrealimentar*

overfeeding—*la sobrealimentación*

oviduct—*el oviducto*

oviducto, el—oviduct

ovinos, los—sheep

owl—*la lechuza, el buho*

owner—*el dueño, la dueña*

ox—*el buey*

P_____

pack (of dogs)—*la jauría*

pad (of a paw)—*la almohadilla plantar*

padecer—to suffer from; *Padece de artitis.*— It suffers from arthritis.

pain—*el dolor*

painfully—*con dolor*

paja, la—straw

la pajarería—pet shop

pájaro, el—bird

pale—*pálido, pálida*

pálido, pálida—pale, pallid

pallid—*pálido, pálida*

palpación, la—palpation

palpar—to palpate

palpate—*palpar*

pant—verb, *jadear*

papada, la—dewlap

parálisis, la—paralysis

paralysis—*la parálisis*

parasites—*los parásitos*

parásitos, los—parasites

pardo, parda—brown; also *marrón* (see *café*)

parvada, la—flock (of chickens)

parvo—*el parvovirus*

parvovirus, el—parvo

parecer—to seem, to appear, to look like

parir—to give birth (used only for animals; for humans, use *dar a luz*)

parrot—*el loro*

parto, el—birth

pasado, pasada—last; *el año pasado*—last year; *la semana pasada*—last week

pasado mañana—day after tomorrow

pasar—to pass, to happen, to occur; *¿Qué le pasó a su animal?*—What happened to your animal?

pastern—*la cuartilla*

pastilla, la—pill

pasto, el—grass, grazing land; *a pasto*— pastured (animals)

pastoreo, el—grazing

pasture—*el pasto*

pastured—*a pasto*; Are they pastured or stabled?—*¿Están a pasto o estabulados?*

pata, la—paw, foot

pato, el, la pata—duck

paw—*la pata*

pedir (i, i)—to ask for

pelear—to fight

pelo, el—fur, pelt

pelt—*el pelo*

pen (stockyard)—*el corral*

pene, el—penis

penis—*el pene*

peor—worse

pequeñas especies, las—small animals

pequeño, pequeña—small (note that "few" or "a little" is *poco*, not *pequeño*)

perder (ie)—to lose

peritonitis—*la peritonitis*

perrera, la—kennel

perro, el, la perra—dog

pesar—to weigh

pescado, el—fish (caught, on a plate); a fish still swimming around is *el pez*

peso, el—weight; *perder peso*—to lose weight; *ganar peso, engordar*—to gain weight

pet—*la mascota*

pet birds—*las aves de jaula*

pet owner—*el dueño, la dueña*

pet shop—*la pajarería*

pez, el—fish (uncaught); *el pescado*—caught fish

pezón, el—teat

pezuña, la—hoof; also, *el casco*

phlegm—*la flema*
physical—*físico, física*
piara, la—herd of pigs
picar—to bite (snakes)
picarse el plumaje—to pluck out its feathers
pico, el—beak
pie, el—foot
piel, la—skin, hide
pierna, la—leg
pig—*el cerdo, la cerda*
pig snare—*la asa trompas*
piglet—*el lechón, la lechona; el cochinillo, la cochinilla*
pigsty—*la pocilga*
pill—*la pastilla*; Give it one of these pills three times a day.—*Dele una de estas pastillas tres veces al día.*
piojos, los—lice
pipa (de girasol), la—sunflower seeds
placenta—*la placenta*
plain—adjective, *sencillo, sencilla*
please—*por favor*
pluck out its feathers—*picarse el plumaje*
pluma, la—feather
plumaje, el—plumage
pneumonia—*la neumonía*; in humans, *la pulmonía*
pocilga, la—pigsty
poco, poca—few; *Tiene pocos defectos.*—It has few defects.; *un poco*—a little; *¿Habla español? Un poco.*—Do you speak Spanish? A little. Note that "small" is *pequeño*, not *poco*.
poder (ue)—to be able to, can (do something), may (do something)
poison—*el veneno*; The goat ate poison.—*La cabra se tragó veneno.*
poll—*la coronilla*
pollito, el, la pollita—chick
polluelo, el, la polluela—chick, baby (pet) birds
polvo, el—powder
poner (an irregular verb)—to put
poner huevos—to lay eggs
poorly—*mal*; The ewe is doing poorly.—*La oveja está mal.*
porcino, porcina—adjective, swine; *la influenza porcina*—swine flu

por favor—please
pork—*el puerco*
porque—because of
possible—*posible*
potranca, la—filly
potranquita, la—foal (female)
potrillo, el—foal (male)
potro, el, la potranca—colt
powder—*el polvo*
precaución, la—precaution, warning (on the label); *como precaución*—as a precaution
precaution—*la precaución*; as a precaution—*como precaución*
pregnant—(use with estar) *gestante* (formal); *preñada* (a little less formal); *cargada* (informal); in humans, *embarazada*
preguntar—to ask (a question)
premios, los—treats (for pets)
prescribe—*recetar*
prescription—*la receta*
presentar—to present; to show signs of
prevenir (ie)—to prevent
prevent—*prevenir* (ie)
prevention—*la prevención, el control*
previo, previa—previous
previous—*previo, previa*
previously—*anteriormente*
prickly pear cactus—*el nopal*
probar (ue)—to prove
problem—*el problema*
problema, el—problem
problematic—*problemático, problemática*
proceder—to proceed
proceed—*proceder*
procrear—to breed
produce—*producir*
producir—to produce
profuse—*profuso, profusa; abundante*
prolapse—*el prolapso*; uterine prolapse—*el prolapso uterino*
pronto—soon, shortly
prove—*probar* (ue)
próximo, próxima—next; *el próximo mes*—next month; *la próxima semana*—next week
prueba, la—test; *los resultados de la prueba*—test results

puerco, el—pork
pulga, la—flea
pulmón, el—lung
pulse—*el pulso*
puppy—*el cachorro, la cachorra; el perrito, la perrita*
purr—*ronronear*
pus—*el pus*; in Mexico, *la pus*
put—*poner* (an irregular verb)

Q

queratitis, la—keratitis
querer (ie)—to want; *quisiera*—I would like. When used with humans, *querer* means "to love."
quince—fifteen
quiste, el—cyst

R

rabbit—*el conejo, la coneja*
rabia, la—rabies
rabies—*la rabia*
rabies control—*el control de la rabia*
rabies vaccine—*la vacuna antirrábica*
rachitic—*raquítico, raquítica*
rachitis—*la raquitis*
ram—*el carnero*
rana, la—frog
rápidamente—rapidly
rapidly—*rápidamente*
raquítico, raquítica—rachitic
raquitis, la—rachitis, rickets
raro, rara—strange, unusual
rascar—to scratch (an itch)
rasp—*escofinar*
raza, la—breed (of animal)
read—*leer*
realizar—to achieve, to carry out. It does not mean "to suddenly understand," which is expressed as *darse cuenta de.*
realize—*darse cuenta de;* I realized that I was wrong.—*Me di cuenta de que estaba equivocado/equivocada.*
rebaño, el—flock (of sheep or goats)
receive—*recibir*
recent—*reciente*
recently—*recientemente, últimamente*

receta, la—prescription
recetar—to prescribe
recibir—to receive
recién nacido, recién nacida—newborn
reciente—recent
recientemente—recently
recomendar (ie)—to recommend
recommend—*recomendar* (ie)
recortar—to cut
recto, el—rectum
rectum—*el recto*
red—*rojo, roja*
reddened—*enrojecido, enrojecida*
reddish—*rojizo, rojiza*
reduce—*reducir, bajar*
reducir—to reduce
refusal to eat—*la aversión por el alimento*
regresar—to come back, to return
relieve (the problem)—*aliviar*
relinchar—to neigh
remediar—to cure
remedio, el—the cure, the remedy
remedy—noun, *el remedio*; verb, *remediar*
remove (a thorn)—*sacar (la espina)*
renal—*renal*
repentino, repentina—sudden
repentinamente—suddenly; also, *de repente*
respiración, la—respiration
respiration—*la respiración*
respirar—to breathe
respiratorio, respiratoria—respiratory
respiratory—*respiratorio, respiratoria*
report (written)—*el informe*
restrain—*sujetar* (for large animals); *sostener* (for small animals) and it is conjugated like *tener*
result—verb, *resultar*; noun, *el resultado*
resultados, los—results (of a test)
results—*los resultados*; test results—*los resultados de la prueba*
reticuloperitonitis traumática, la—hardware disease
return, come back—*volver* (ue), *regresar*
review (test results)—*revisar*
revisar—to go over (test results), to check over
rhinoceros—*el rinoceronte*
rickets—*la raquitis*

rid, get rid of—*expulsar (parásitos)*
rider (of horses)—*el jinete, la jinete*
rigid—*rígido, rígida*
rigidez, la—rigidity
rigidity—*la rigidez*
rígido, rígida—rigid
rinoceronte, el—rhinoceros
riñón, el—kidney
rodilla, la—knee
rojizo, rojiza—reddish
rojo, roja—red
romperse—to break; *Se le rompió la pierna.*—It broke its leg.
ronronear—to purr
rooster—*el gallo*
ruido, el—noise, sound
rumen—*el rumen*
ruminant—noun, *el rumiante*; adjective, *rumiante*
ruminate—*rumiar*
rump—*la grupa*
run (not walk)—*correr*
run over—*atropellar*; It was run over by a car.—*Le atropelló un auto.*
rut, season—*celo*; The animal is in season.—*Está en celo.*
ryegrass—*el ballico*

S_____
sábado, el—Saturday
sacar—to remove (a thorn)
sacudir—to shake (head or horns)
sal, la—salt
sala de espera, la—waiting room
salegar, la—salt lick, salt block
saliva—*la saliva*
salivar—to salivate
salivate—*salivar*
salt—*la sal*
salt lick, salt block—*la salegar*
sample—*la muestra*; stool sample—*las muestras de excremento*
sangrar—to bleed
sangre, la—blood
sanguiolento, sanguiolenta—bloody
sarna, la—mange; *el antisárnico*—antimange remedy

Saturday—*el sábado*
scant—*escaso, escasa; poco, poca*
science—*la ciencia*
scraps, table scraps, leftovers—*las sobras (de comida)*
scratch—(with itching) *rascar*; (with claws to draw blood) *arañar*
scrotum—*el escroto*
season—*el celo*; The animal is in season—*Está en celo.*
seco, seca—dry
secreción, la—secretion
sedum—*la hierba callera*
seeds—*las semillas*
seem—*parecer*; to show signs of—*mostrar (ue), presentar*
seguir (i, i)—to continue, to keep on; *Siga el tratamiento*—Continue the treatment; *Siga dándole los suplementos*—Keep giving it the supplements.
seis—six
seizures—*las convulsiones*
self-sufficient—*autosuficiente*
sell—*vender*
semana, la—week; *la próxima semana*—next week; *la semana pasada*—last week
semillas, las—seeds
sencillo, sencilla—simple, uncomplicated
separado, separada—isolated
separar—to isolate
septic—*séptico, séptica*
septicemia, la—septicemia; blood poisoning
séptico, séptica—septic
ser (an irregular verb)—to be (used with personality traits or physical characteristics or profession); *La señora Rodríguez es simpática. El perro es negro. Yo soy veterinaria*—Mrs. Rodríguez is nice. The dog is black. I am a veterinarian.
serie, la—series
series—*la serie*
serious—*serio, seria; grave*
serpiente, la—snake; also *la culebra*
seven—*siete*
sex—*el sexo*; gender—*el género*
sexo, el—sex; *el género*—gender

shake—*sacudir* (head or horns); *temblar*
(ie)—tremble, shiver

shank—*la caña*

shark—*el tiburón*

sheep—*los ovinos, las ovejas, el ganado
lanar*

shell—*el caparazón* (turtle); *la cáscara*
(egg)

shiver—*temblar* (ie)

shivering—*los temblores*

shoot—*disparar;* The hunter shot it.—*El
cazador le disparó.*

shortly—*pronto;* I'll be with you shortly—
Estaré con usted pronto.

shot—*la inyección* (injection); *el disparo* (gun)

should—*deber*

shoulder—*el hombro*

show signs of—*mostrar* (ue), *presentar*

shrink—*disminuir*

sick—*enfermo, enferma;* (seriously) *mórbido,
mórbida; grave*

sickness—*la enfermedad*

siete—seven

signo, el—sign, symptom

siguiente—following; *la siguiente manera*—
the following manner

silage—*el ensilaje*

simpático, simpática—nice, personable (only
for humans, not for objects)

simple—*sencillo, sencilla*

síntoma, el—symptom

sistema, el—system; *el sistema nervioso*—
nervous system

situation—*la situación*

six—*seis*

skin—*la piel*

sleep—*dormir* (ue, u)

slowly—*despacio, lentamente;* Speak more
slowly, please.—*Hable más despacio, por
favor.*

small—*pequeño, pequeña; chiquito, chiquita*

small animals—*las pequeñas especies*

smell—noun, *el olor;* verb, *oler* (ue); It
smells bad.—*Huele mal.;* to give off a
bad smell—*dar mal olor;* (sense of
smell) *el olfato*

smelly—*fétido, fétida; huele mal*

snake—*la culebra, la serpiente*

sobras, las—table scraps, leftovers

sobrealimentar—to overfeed

solución, la—solution

solution—(to a problem) *la solución;*
(dissolved in liquid) *la disolución*

someter—to subject (to tests, examination);
to undergo

so much—*tanto, tanta*

sonido, el—sound, noise

soon—*pronto*

sordera, la—deafness

sordo, sorda—deaf

sore (ulcer)—noun, *la llaga*

sorghum—*el sorgo*

sorgo, el—sorghum

sostener (conjugated like *tener*)—to hold
still (a small animal; use *sujetar* with a
large animal)

sound, noise—*el sonido*

sow—*la cerda*

spay—*capar, castrar*

spayed—*capado, capada; castrado, castrada*

speak—*hablar*

specialist—*el especialista, la especialista*

species—*la especie*

sporadic—*esporádico, esporádica; de vez en
cuando; a veces*

spotted (with blood)—*manchado,
manchada (de sangre)*

squirt—*introducir;* Squirt this in its
mouth.—*Introduzca esto por la boca.*

stable—noun, *el establo;* adjective, *estable*

stabled (animals)—*estabulado, estabulada*

stagger—verb, *tambalearse*

staggers—noun, *el vértigo*

stall—*la caseta, la caballeriza*

stallion—*el semental, el garañón*

stand up—*levantarse*

start—noun, *el comienzo;* verb, *comenzar*
(ie); *empezar* (ie)

steer—*el novillo*

sterile—*estéril; infecundo, infecunda; infértil*

still, yet—*todavía;* Lucky still doesn't have
arthritis—*Lucky todavía no tiene artritis;*
hold still—*sujetar, sostener*

stillbirth—*el mortinato*

stockyard—*el corral*

stomach—*el estómago*

stool—*el excremento*; stool sample—*las muestras de excremento*

strange, odd—*extraño, extraña*

straw—*la paja*

stream (of urine)—*el chorro*

subir—to rise, to go up

subject (to tests)—*someter*

suceder—to occur, to happen

sudden—*repentino, repentina*

suddenly—*repentinamente, de repente*

suffer—*sufrir*; suffer from—*padecer de*

sufficient—*suficiente*

suficiente—sufficient

sufrir—to suffer

sugerir (ie, i)—to suggest

suggest—*sugerir* (ie, i)

sujetar—restrain, hold still (large animal); use *sostener* with a small animal

Sunday—*el domingo*

sunflower seeds—*la pipa (de girasol)*

sunken—*hundido, hundida*

suplementos, los—supplements

supplements—*los suplementos*

supurar—to discharge (with pus)

surgery—*la cirugía*

swallow—*tragar*

swell—*hinchar; inflamar*

swelling—*el hinchazón* (informal); *la tumefacción* (formal)

swine—noun, *el ganado porcino, los cerdos*; adjective, *porcino, porcina*; herd of swine—*la piara*

swine flu—*la influenza porcina*

swollen—*hinchado, hinchada; inflamado, inflamada*

symptom—*el síntoma* (if the phenomenon can't be measured, such as pain); *el signo* (if the phenomenon can be measured, such as fever)

system—*el sistema*

systematic—*sistemático, sistemática*

T

table scraps, leftovers—*las sobras (de comida)*

tail—*la cola*

take—(care of) *cuidar de*; (temperature) *tomar*; (biopsy) *sacar*

talon—*la garra*

talón, el—heel

también—also

tame, docile—*manso, mansa*

tanto, tanta—so much

tapeworm—*la lombriz*

tarso, el—hock

teary—*lloroso, llorosa*

teat—*el pezón; la teta*

teat dipping—*el enjuage de los pezones*

tejido, el—tissue

tell—*decir* (an irregular verb)

temblar (ie)—to shake, to tremble

temblores, los—trembling; the shakes

temperatura, la—temperature; *tomar la temperatura*—to take its temperature.

temperature—*la temperatura*; I'm going to take its temperature.—*Voy a tomar su temperatura.*

ten—*diez*

tend—(custom) *tender* (ie); It tends to fall down.—*Tiende a caerse*; take care of—*cuidar de*; The owner takes good care of his sheep.—*El dueño cuida bien de sus ovejas.*

tendencia, la—tendency

tendency—*la tendencia*

tender (ie)—to tend to; *Tiende a caerse*—It tends to fall down.

tener (an irregular verb)—to have, to own; *tener que* + infinitive—to have to (do something)

tenue—faint, weak

terapéutico, terapéutica,—therapeutic

terapia, la—therapy

terminar—to finish (a task)

termómetro, el—thermometer

ternero, el, la ternera—calf

test—*la prueba*; test results—*los resultados de la prueba*

testicle—*el testículo*

testículo, el—testicle

teta, la—teat

tetania, la—tetany

tétanos, el—tetanus

tetanus—*el tétanos;* tetanus shot—*el antitetánico*

tetany—*la tetania*

therapy—*la terapia*

therapeutic—*terapéutico, terapéutica*

there is, there are—*hay* (pronounced like "eye")

thermometer—*el termómetro*

thick—*espeso, espesa*

thin—*flaco, flaca* (informal); *delgado, delgada* (formal); (thin liquid) *tenue, fluido, fluida*

think, believe—*creer;* I think it has anemia—*Creo que tiene anemia.*

this—*este, esta;* this afternoon—*esta tarde;* this month—*este mes;* this morning—*esta mañana;* this week—*esta semana*

thorax—*el tórax*

thorn—*la espina;* It has a thorn in its paw—*Tiene espina en la pata.*

three—*tres*

Thursday—*el jueves*

tiburón, el—shark

tick—*la garrapata;* ixodid ticks—*las garrapatas ixodes*

tiger—*el tigre*

tigre, el—tiger

time (hours, minutes)—*el tiempo*

times (occurences)—*las veces;* at times—*a veces;* three times a day—*tres veces al día*

timpanizado, timpanizada—bloated

tinged (with blood)—*manchado, manchada (de sangre)*

tire—*cansar;* to tire easily—*cansar fácilmente*

tissue—*el tejido*

todavía—still, yet; *Lucky todavía no tiene artritis.*—Lucky doesn't have arthritis yet.

today—*hoy*

todos los días—every day

toe—*el dedo*

tomar—to drink, to take (temperature, x-rays)

tomorrow—*mañana;* tomorrow afternoon—*mañana por la tarde;* tomorrow morning—*mañana por la mañana*

tonight—*esta noche*

too, too much—*demasiado, demasiada*

tórax, el—thorax

toro, el—bull

torta, la—cake; *la torta de algodón*—cottonseed cake; *la torta oleaginosa*—oil cake

tos, la—cough

toser—to cough

toxemia—*la toxemia*

toxic—*tóxico, tóxica*

toxicity—*la toxicidad*

tóxico, tóxica—toxic

toxin—*la toxina*

toxina, la—toxin

trabajar—to work

trabajo, el—noun, work, job

trachea—*la tráquea*

tragar—to swallow; *Se tragó un clavo.*—It swallowed a nail.

tráquea, la—trachea

tratamiento, el—treatment

tratar—to treat (a patient*); tratar de +* infinitive—to try (to do something)

treat (a patient)—*tratar*

treats (for pets)—*las galletitas, los premios, las botanas, los obsequios*

treatment—*el tratamiento*

trébol, el—clover

tremble—*temblar* (ie)

trembling—noun, *los temblores*

tres—three

tripa, la—intestine

trot—*trotar*

trotar—to trot

try—noun, *el esfuerzo;* verb, *tratar de +* infinitive; I try to speak Spanish.—*Trato de hablar español.*

Tuesday—*el martes*

tumbado, tumbada—lying down

tumor—*el tumor*

turbio, turbia—cloudy, with sediment; *La orina está turbia*—The urine is cloudy.

twelve—*doce*
twice—*dos veces*
two—*dos*

U

ubre, la—udder
udder—*la ubre*
ulcer—*la úlcera, la llaga*
últimamente—lately, recently
un, uno, una—one, a; *un día*—one day, a
  day; *¿Cuántos tumores tiene? Sólo uno*—
  How many tumors does it have? Just
  one; *una semana*—one week, a week
undergo (testing, treatment)—*someter*
understand—*comprender*
ungüento, el—ointment
until—*hasta*
unusual—*raro, rara; extraño, extraña*
uña, la—nail, toenail
urinate—*orinar*
urine—*la orina*
útero, el—uterus
uterus—*el útero*
urinary bladder—*la vesícula urinaria*
use—noun, *el uso*; verb, *usar, utilizar*
uso, el—use
utilizar—to use

V

vaca, la—cow; *las vacas lecheras*—dairy
  cows
vacío, vacío—empty
vaccinate—*vacunar*
vaccinations—*las vacunas*
vacuna, la—vaccine; *la vacuna
  antirrábica*—rabies vaccine
vacunar—to vaccinate
vagina—*la vagina*
vaquilla, la—heifer
veces, las—times, occurrences; three times
  a day—*tres veces al día; a veces*—at
  times
vegetables—*las verduras*; fresh vegetables—
  las verduras frescas
vein—*la vena*
vejiga, la—urinary bladder
vena yugular, la—jugular vein

venado, el—deer
venda, la—bandage
vendajes, los—bandages
vendar—to bandage
vender—to sell
veneno, el—poison; *Se tragó el veneno.*—It
  drank poison.
verde—green
verduras, las—vegetables; *las verduras
  frescas*—fresh vegetables
verraco, el—boar
vértigo, el—vertigo; staggers
very—*muy*
vesícula, la—bladder; *la vesícula biliar*—gall
  bladder; *la vesícula urinaria*—urinary
  bladder
vetch—*la veza*
veterinarian—noun, *el veterinario, la
  veterinaria*; adjective, *veterinario,
  veterinaria*
veterinario, veterinaria—noun, veterinarian;
  adjective, veterinary
vez, la—time (occurence); *una vez*—one
  time, once; *dos veces*—two times
la veza—vetch
viernes, el—Friday
virus—*el virus*
vitamin—*la vitamina*; vitamin C—*la
  vitamina C*; vitamin C deficiency—*la
  carencia de la vitamina C*
vitamina, la—vitamin
vivir—to live
volar (ue)—to fly
volver (ue)—to return
vomit—verb, *vomitar*; noun, *el vómito*
vomitar—to vomit
vómito, el—noun, vomit, vomiting
vulva—*la vulva*

W

wait—*esperar, aguardar;* Wait a moment,
  please.—*Espere un momento, por favor;*
  Please wait in the waiting room.—*Por
  favor, aguarde en la sala de espera.*
waiting room—*la sala de espera*
walk—*caminar, marchar;* to walk in
  circles—*marchar en círculos*

want—*querer* (ie)
warnings (on the label)—*las precauciones (en la etiqueta)*
wash—*lavar*
wasp—*la avispa*
watch, observe—*observar*
water—*el agua*
water dish, water trough—*el bebedero*
watery, teary—*lloroso, llorosa*
watery milk—*la leche acuosa*
weak—*débil*
wean—*destetar*
weaned—*destetado, destetada*
weaning—*el destete*
Wednesday—*el miércoles*
week—*la semana*
weigh—*pesar;* It weighs ten kilos.—*Pesa diez kilos.*
weight—*el peso;* to lose weight—*perder* (ie) *peso;* to gain weight—*ganar peso, engordar*
wet food—*la comida húmeda*
wether—*el carnero capado*
whale—*la ballena*
What?—*¿Qué?*
what's best—*lo mejor*
when—*cuando, ¿Cuándo?*
where—*donde, ¿Dónde?*
white—*blanco, blanca*
wife—*la esposa*
wing—*el ala, las alas*
wire—*el alambre;* barbed wire—*el alambre de púas;* electrical wire—*el cable eléctrico*
withers—*la cruz*
wool—*la lana*

worm—noun, *el gusano, la lombriz;* verb, *desparasitar*
worse—*peor*
worsen—*empeorar*
wound, injury—*la herida*
write—*escribir;* this verb is regular except in the present perfect: *he escrito*

X

x-ray—*los rayos x* (pronounced "ECKees"; the letter itself is called *equis*); to take an x-ray—*tomar unos rayos x*

Y

ya—already
year—*el año* (caution: not *el ano*, which is "anus")
yegua, la—mare
yellow—*amarillo, amarilla.* If the color is natural, use with *ser;* The canary is yellow.—*El canario es amarillo.* If the color is a condition, use with *estar;* Its eyes are yellow.—*Los ojos están amarillos.*
yellowish—*amarillento, amarillenta*
yerba, la—grass
yesterday—*ayer;* yesterday afternoon—*ayer por la tarde;* last night—*anoche*
yet—*todavía;* Lucky doesn't have arthritis yet—*Lucky todavía no tiene artritis.*
yodo, el—iodine

Z

zanahoria, la—carrot
zebra—*la cebra*
zorro, el—fox